PRAISE FOR
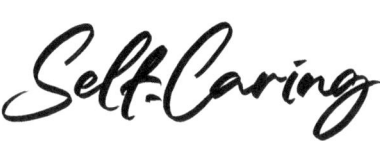

"*Self-Caring* is a masterclass in caring for yourself. It's powerfully packed with proven strategies for creating a new path toward well-being and inner peace. Michelle Peck has spent decades honoring, teaching, and studying the science and art of caring, and now her brilliant hands-on book offers innovative, proven, and yet simple practices that will help you accomplish more by actually doing less. No matter who and where you are in life, I promise you will benefit from this book. It's THAT good!"

—**JACK CANFIELD**, *Co-author of the bestselling Chicken Soup for the Soul® Series and a pioneer in the fields of personal development and peak performance*

"*Self-Caring* is a practical masterpiece. Michelle Peck not only tells the reader how to create a self-fulfilling prophecy of wellness and happiness, but she also provides an experiential, highly inspiring guide for achieving this. Through her Gratitude Journal and Healthy-Habit Workbook, she helps you turn your dreams into realities."

—**GEORGE S. EVERLY, JR., PhD**, *Co-founder of The International Critical Incident Stress Foundation and author of* Leading Beyond Crisis *and* The Johns Hopkins Guide to Psychological First Aid

"Wow! What a fabulous gift to the world! *Self-Caring* is nothing less than a catalyst for falling in love with yourself and life! If you know you need to pause and take stock, if you want more balance and joy, this book will help you live, learn, grow, and bless yourself (and others) along the way. Every page and word are imbued with Universal Love."

—JEAN WATSON, PhD, RN, AHN-BC, FAAN, LL (AAN), *Founder, Watson Caring Science Institute; Distinguished Professor/Dean Emerita, University of Colorado, Denver, College of Nursing*

"Michelle Peck's *Self-Caring* provides a path for discovering how to use and grow your inner resources. This beautifully structured book, grounded in Caring Science and self-reflection, guides you to look inward, nurture, and holistically care for yourself. Even if you've been on a self-improvement path for decades, there's something essential for you in this book."

—SARA HORTON-DEUTSCH, PhD, RN, FAAN, ANEF, *Caritas Coach®, Director, University of San Francisco/Kaiser Permanente Partnership; Professor, University of San Francisco School of Nursing and Health Professions*

"Drawing on years of devoted study, teaching, and caring for people, Michelle guides readers on a transformational and straight-forward path to well-being.

This brilliantly balanced book makes listening to our hearts, maximizing our inner resources, and living our highest and best potential accessible, practical, achievable, and easy to understand."

—LINH NGUYEN, MD, MEd, EdD, *Associate Professor, McGovern Medical School at UTHealth Houston, Hospice and Palliative Medicine*

"Michelle is the perfect guide for us all on the journey of self-caring. When you read this book, you won't feel like you're reading a book but more like you stepped through a portal onto a path of self-reflection, wisdom, compassion, and so much more. Michelle inspires us to embrace joy-affirming habits that open our hearts and nurture our well-being. Her seven-step guidebook provides uplifting stories, mystic poetry, intentional journaling, and, most importantly, a proven and practical structure—equally empowering for those of us new to self-caring and for those looking to enhance and expand our journey. By the last page of this amazing book, you will emerge with a stronger sense of wellness through the strength of inner love."

—LEE REVERE, PhD, *Professor, University of Florida, College of Public Health and Health Professions, Health Services Research, Management and Policy*

Self-Caring

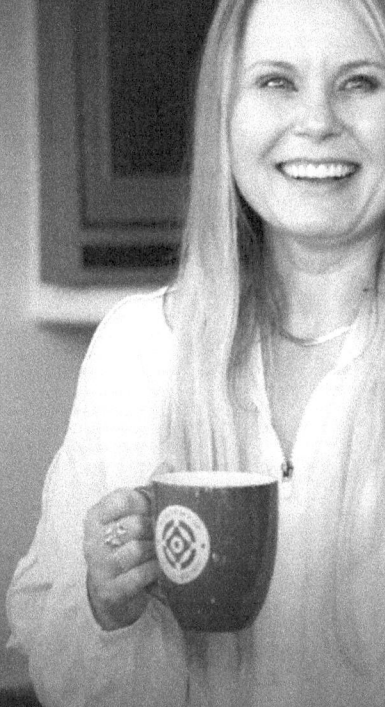

with
MINDFUL GRATITUDE JOURNAL
plus
HEALTHY-HABIT WORKBOOK

A WELL-BEING GUIDEBOOK
MICHELLE PECK

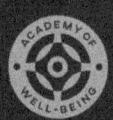

Copyright © 2022 by Michelle Peck

All rights reserved.

Published in the United States

Academy of Well-Being, LLC, Conroe, Texas

academyofwellbeing.com

This book is the property of Michelle Peck. No part of this book may be reproduced, stored within a retrieval system, or transmitted in any form or by any means without the author's written permission.

Hardcover ISBN: 979-8-9860479-0-4

Paperback ISBN: 979-8-9860479-1-1

E-book ISBN: 979-8-9860479-2-8

Printed in the United States of America

Cover design and photography by Joss Cast

Cover production and interior design by Marisa Jackson

Edited by Peter Lundell and Sage Taylor Kingsley

Contact team@academyofwellbeing.com

*To Raul, Leon,
Nico, Linh,
the companion dogs,
and all who brighten humanity
by embracing self-growth
and well-being along their
caring journey.*

DISCLAIMER

This book contains advice and information related to wellness, self-growth, and caring for yourself. It should supplement and not replace the advice of your health professionals. You are advised to consult your health professionals about matters related to your health and issues that may require diagnosis or medical attention. All efforts have been made to ensure the accuracy of the information in this book as of the date of publication. The publisher and author disclaim liability for any medical outcomes due to applying or failing to apply the methods suggested in this book. Although every effort has been made to ensure that the personal and professional advice presented within this book is useful and appropriate, the author and publisher do not assume and hereby disclaim any liability to any person choosing to employ the guidance offered in this book.

This is a work of creative non-fiction. All the events are accurate to the best of the author's memory. Names and identifying features have been changed to protect the identity of certain parties.

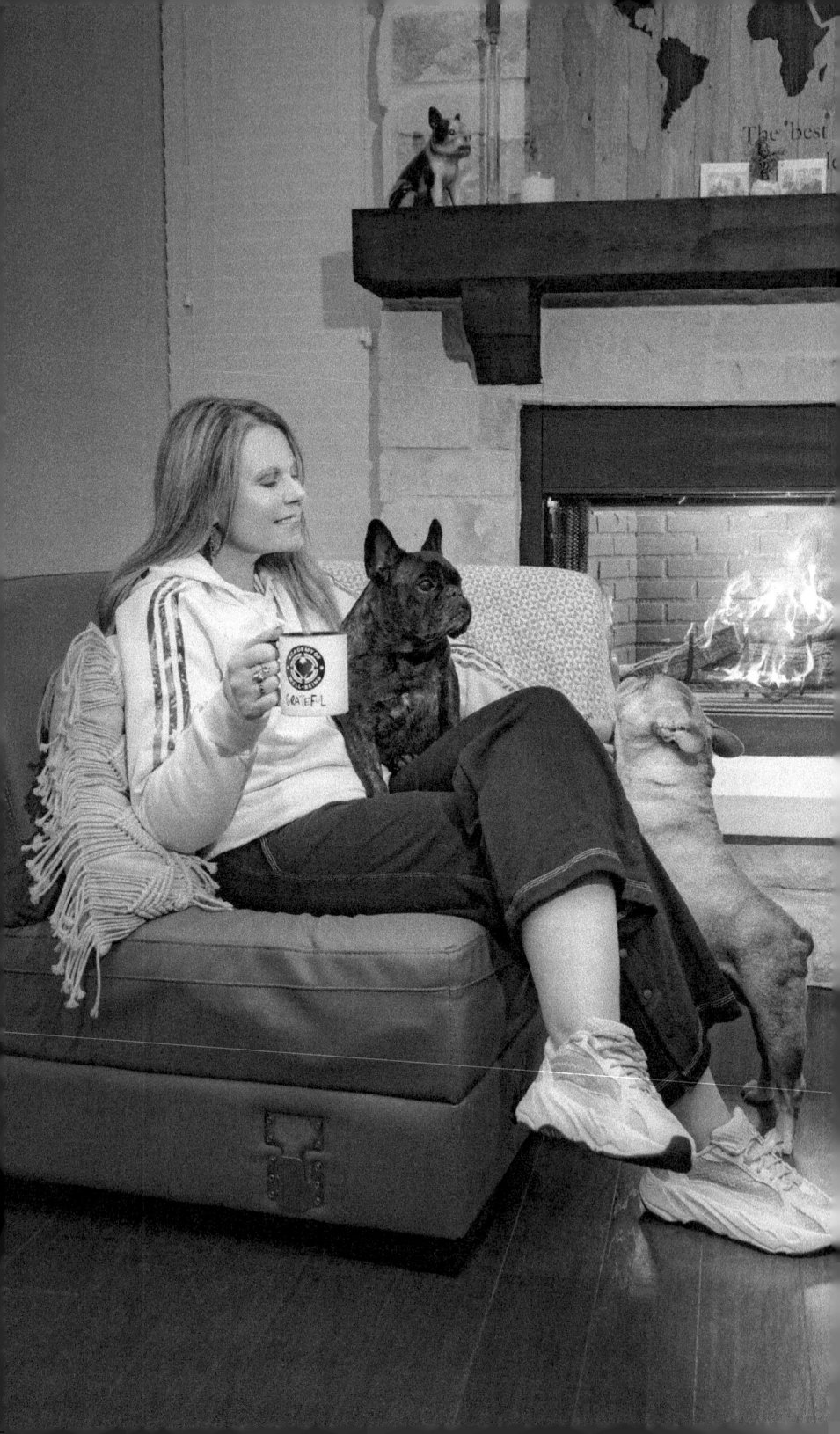

Welcome

WELCOME TO SELF-CARING!

Self-Caring takes us on a journey to optimize our well-being, self-growth, and caring potential. As we strengthen our awareness, we will pay more attention to the present moment, live based on what is here and now, align with nature, and easily incorporate self-care practices into our lifestyle. This book is designed to help us self-discover, reflect, and learn techniques to improve our physical, mental, emotional, and spiritual wellness.

For the 7-Step Mindful Gratitude Journal and Healthy-Habit Workbook sections, I recommend typing or writing your responses on a blank sheet or using the pages provided. The lines here are intended to capture whatever you feel needs to be said in response to each question. It is also okay to delete your work or throw out pages; this symbolizes moving forward. If

SELF-CARING

you purchased this book in an electronic format and desire printable journal/workbook pages, you can find them at www.academyofwellbeing.com (or use the QR code on the next page).

Caring for ourselves should never leave us feeling selfish or guilty—it is a requirement for reaching our highest and best well-being, self-growth, and caring potential. I hope that you will allow yourself to free your emotions when they surface and not store them in your physiology. Also, our past should not hold us in prison. Life is about growing from lessons, not serving life sentences.

Here's an example of how to use the Intention and Plan sections.

INTENTION:

Whenever *I start reaching for junk food* **(situation arises), I will respond by** *sipping a full glass of water before committing to my choice*

I can ask for anything. What am I asking the Universe for?
To be full of energy and shine my light on the world

WELCOME

OPTIMIZING PLAN:

I will do *a guided meditation*
for this amount of time: *15 minutes*
in this place: *my meditation room*
starting *this Saturday* **and**
repeating every *morning at 7:00 am*

IF-THEN PLAN:

If *my morning meditation gets interrupted*
then I will remain flexible and instead
do my meditation before lunch

Using heart-centering techniques, healthy habits, mindful gratitude journaling, affirmations, intentions, and plans will help us move forward and grow on our paths. So now is our time to open our hearts and minds. I wish you all the best. I'm happy that we're here together!

In gratitude,

Michelle

Contents

Foreword *Sage Taylor Kingsley*	*xvii*

PART I   ASPIRE   *1*

Getting Started	*3*
Aspire & Upgrade Our Systems	*15*
Meet Our Guide	*21*
Mindful Gratitude Journal Step 1: Aspire	*27*
Healthy-Habit Workbook Step 1: Aspire	*35*

PART II   BELONGING   *41*

Unlock the Door of Belonging	*43*
Mindful Gratitude Journal Step 2: Wholeness	*51*
Healthy-Habit Workbook Step 2: Wholeness	*55*
Step Through the Doorway of Belonging	*59*
Mindful Gratitude Journal Step 3: Courage	*71*
Healthy-Habit Workbook Step 3: Courage	*79*

Belonging Before Being, Knowing & Doing *83*

    Mindful Gratitude Journal · *Step 4: Belonging* *93*

    Healthy-Habit Workbook · *Step 4: Belonging* *101*

PART III · WELL-BEING *105*

The History of Caring *107*

Embrace Ourselves *113*

    Mindful Gratitude Journal · *Step 5: Embrace* *125*

    Healthy-Habit Workbook · *Step 5: Embrace* *131*

Inspire & Jump Again *135*

Gratitude, Balance & Energy in Motion *145*

    Mindful Gratitude Journal · *Step 6: Balance* *151*

    Healthy-Habit Workbook · *Step 6: Balance* *159*

Well-Being, We Are Blooming *163*

    Mindful Gratitude Journal · *Step 7: Blooming* *169*

    Healthy-Habit Workbook · *Step 7: Blooming* *179*

About the Author *185*

Endnotes *187*

Foreword

Let our first words
from pen and lips
be: "Thank you"
be: "I love you"
be: "I am blessed."
The day embraces us
as we embrace the day.

SAGE

Since 1994, I've had the joy of serving as a spiritual teacher, healer, and messenger, creating dozens of courses and facilitating re-Treats and sessions on many self-growth subjects, including self-love.

I've also recently had the privilege of serving as editor and proofreader for *Self-Caring*, which is how Michelle Peck and

I connected. We instantly recognized one another as kindred spirits. So when Michelle asked me to write this "Foreword," I felt excited and delighted.

Love and caring are imbued into every page of this extraordinary book, and it is my honor to recommend it.

Most kind-hearted people have a tendency to give so much that we become depleted. We all have heard the "put the oxygen mask on yourself first" analogy, but in real life, when our loved ones have needs, expectations, and demands, it's not always easy to find a balance between caring for them and caring for ourselves. Michelle's book helps us rediscover how vital it really is to care for ourselves and how to recommit to making self-caring a way of life.

Self-caring is the action aspect of self-love.

And caring for ourselves is not just a good idea; it's essential. The good news is: When we get more masterful at self-caring, we can actually make an even BIGGER difference because we can give and serve from an overflowing cup.

In my work with people worldwide, I have seen that the number-one issue everyone has is the need to love themselves —and their lives—much more.

FOREWORD

More freely.

More deeply.

More playfully.

More consistently.

More unconditionally.

And much more joyously.

THIS book is much more than a book. It's a pathway home to ourselves and

> … To enhancing our relationships with others by caring more for ourselves.
>
> … To creating more balance, flow, ease, and grace.
>
> … And to remembering who we truly are.

Michelle has beautifully woven together:

1. Empowering exercises that will both soothe and uplift us instantly.
2. Real examples of how greater self-caring changes lives, hearts, and the world.

3. Insightful questions for self-reflection and greater connection with what truly sources us and makes us come alive.
4. Simple yet effective ways to build better habits to enhance our well-being.
5. Tips, tools, and teachings for living with more gratitude and peace every day.
6. Messages of love and highest truth from Sufi poet Rumi.

Michelle's personal and professional experience—as a nurse, coach, an expert certified in numerous self-caring-oriented modalities, and as a loving mother, wife, dog mom, and human BE-ing—all have prepared her to gorgeously gestate Self-Caring into the world.

And please know that *Self-Caring* is not just another "shelf-help" book to buy, skim, set, and forget. This is a gift to ourselves from ourselves that keeps on giving, so, please go slowly here, go wide, go deep.

Savor and be nourished.

Receive.

When Michelle asked her intuition who should write this "Foreword," she received a message: "Sage should write it

FOREWORD

because she writes like Rumi." The amazing thing is that, at the time, Michelle had had no idea that I am also a mystic poet, in a similar style to Rumi sometimes (on a really good day).

So, in the spirit of Rumi, may I share a poem to bless this new beginning here?

Taking care
Taking care of the home
Taking care of everyone
Taking care of the breath
Taking care of the rhythm
Taking care of the balance
Taking care of the creatures
Taking care of the mind's thirst
Taking care of the fingers' itches
Taking care of the body's temple
Taking care of the passion's ache
Taking care of the eyes' longing for beauty
Taking care of the ears' need for silence and birdsong
Taking care of the skin's yearning for touch
Taking care to walk lightly on the Earth
Taking care of the soul's hunger
Taking care of the self
Taking care

SAGE

SELF-CARING

As Rumi would perhaps say to us all:

Beloved, you deserve every blessing.

You were guided to this right now for a reason. Please celebrate your self-caring choice and immerse in the delightful bliss bath that is this book…

—Rev. Sage Taylor Kingsley, B.A., CHT, Reiki Master, editor, copywriter, and mystic poet at SageforYourPage.com; international best-selling co-author of *Embraced by the Divine* and *Feisty: Dangerously Amazing Women Using Their Voices & Making an Impact*

Seek the wisdom
that will untie your knot.
Seek the path
that demands your
whole being.

RUMI

· PART I ·

Aspire

Yesterday I was clever,
so I wanted to change the world.
Today I am wise, so I am changing myself.

RUMI

Come, come,
whoever you are.
Wanderer, worshiper, lover
of leaving. It doesn't matter.
Ours is not a caravan of despair.
Come, even if you have broken
your vows a thousand
times. Come, yet again,
come, come.

RUMI

Getting Started

*Have you ever thought,
there has to be a better way?*

Launching my first company was exhilarating, but only two years into my consulting practice, my health suffered. I lived with fatigue, digestion issues, rashes, headaches, back pain, and trouble sleeping. Although I was productive and successful, I knew something had to change. One morning in the spring of 2009, I rushed into work late, thanks to waiting in the long line at the coffee shop, where I fueled up multiple times a day. When I finally arrived, I placed my jumbo black coffee and energy drink down on one end of the table and looked across the long conference room table. I was terrified. Four out of ten of my nursing students were drinking the same jumbo-sized energy drink I was. I felt disappointed and discouraged about the role model I had become.

SELF-CARING

A few months later I was doing rounds with a physician I'll call Doc. And something happened that changed my life forever. My heartbeat was irregular, and Doc's advice was to start wearing a heart monitor. Seriously. I was only in my early thirties, and this was more than I wanted to cope with.

As a nurse practitioner caring for older adults, I knew all the recipes—treatments, medications, diagnoses, and workups.

I also knew that my symptoms stacking up were leading to a life filled with more discomforts and hurts. I already needed to take stomach acid blockers multiple times a day, and the coughing from my irritated digestive tract was almost unbearable. Now my heart was skipping beats.

A few months later, another 7 a.m. rounds session with Doc. I was so desperate to feel better that I made a deal. In exchange for all the stomach acid blockers stored in Doc's supply room, I would help him write out every note and write all the orders he needed as he treated patients that day. I felt victorious that afternoon as I carried a huge box with hundreds of small sample bottles to my car. But as I opened each tiny bottle one by one and counted the capsules while dropping them into a large bottle, I felt guilty and cringed. Was this how my life would be?

These defining moments forced me to look for a better way.

GETTING STARTED

After four years of running a successful company, my body was tired and sore. As I rested my throbbing, aching forehead on my office desk, the cold surface was soothing. Closing my eyes allowed me to visualize what life would be like five years from now if everything went according to plan. But then tears filled my eyes and streamed onto the desk. I realized that my work was not worth the pain it caused me. Fear took over as visions of disease filled my mind. My death approached if things didn't change soon. I took a deep breath and rested. I began to feel calm in the stillness. Then something unexpected happened. An updated version of my future showed up, including a house surrounded by nature with dogs on my lap, a spouse, and children waiting for me.

I felt encouraged and decided to take control of my life.

Fortunately, I grew up around my grandfather, a gracious listener and orthopedic surgeon, who told me countless stories about recovery. So I knew from an early age that there were more than treatments. Healing was an option. As a child, I doubted my grandfather's insight when he said that one of the biggest problems with modern medicine was too much specialization. But during my new client visits, his wisdom resonated deeply in my heart when the numbers of medicines, diagnoses, and specialists were often too many to count.

SELF-CARING

I also have been an avid reader throughout my life. As a teenager, I began turning to books to solve everyday challenges. I never have enjoyed problems, but solutions are my specialty. As I turned to the colored drawings in the center of Bernie Siegal's *Love Medicine & Miracles,* they revealed an inner knowingness about disease and healing potential.[1] Many people have wanted to buy this book after hearing me read just one story from the yellowed and worn pages.

Like Siegal, I was privileged to meet many exceptional patients during my clinical nursing practice. Repeatedly, they taught me to consider wholeness over the sum of parts. I also learned to unguard and open my heart when they and their family members expressed love while I cared for them.

Enough is enough. I would heal myself.

By 2011, I'd had enough and set out on a mission to heal myself and help others do the same. I read, researched, tried different remedies, and learned that our bodies are much more intelligent than we think. In addition, emotions, thoughts, and physical surroundings impact our overall well-being (optimal experience and functioning). The answers are not as simple as eating better or exercising more; they are about understanding yourself completely and addressing the root causes of symptoms.

GETTING STARTED

I got to the roots of my symptoms and healed.

After healing, I began teaching these new well-being, self-growth, and caring ways and dedicated myself to lifelong learning. I became a Watson Caring Science Institute-Certified Caritas Coach® and discovered how my healing experience aligned with the scientific field of Caring Science. Then as a Chopra Health™ and Chopra Meditation™ Instructor, I found how my experience aligned with modern science and the science of life (Ayurvedic medicine). Experiencing my healing, Self-Caring transformation, and teaching these new ways of well-being, self-growth, and caring have been the most rewarding moments of my twenty-plus years in nursing.

Our world is stressful, chaotic, and exhausting. We all want to be happy, healthy, and productive, but we often hold on to limiting beliefs that keep us stuck. For years I was frustrated with my life while knowing there had to be a better way. What I learned from the path leading to my Self-Caring Revival, coupled with decades of studying, teaching, and caring for thousands of people, was that what worked for me also was helping others shift their lives as well.

Self-Caring means fueling up from the inside.

SELF-CARING

Self-Caring means growing and caring for our inner selves. Caring for ourselves is foundational and comes before compassionately caring for other people. Unfortunately, most of us are not taught this way of caring in school. As a result, we often suffer when we could be enjoying life more fully. This book will help us awaken, use, and grow our inner resources.

Tremendous power is inside this book and inside all of us!

This book will help us get unstuck. We will remedy racing thoughts and toxic negative thinking cycles by practicing these techniques. Living life with balance, success, and happiness becomes more accessible and natural as we learn to use and grow our inner resources. The knowledge contained in this power-packed book has helped countless people transform their lives to start living happier.

This book combines a seven-step method with five elements. The seven steps are: (1) Aspire, (2) Wholeness, (3) Courage, (4) Belonging, (5) Embrace, (6) Balance, and (7) Blooming.

The five elements are: (1) Story and Science, (2) Heart-Centering Techniques, (3) Mindful Gratitude Journal, (4) Healthy-Habit Workbook and Plans, and (5) Intention and Affirmation.

GETTING STARTED

1. STORY AND SCIENCE

There is no doubt that stories and science are both potent tools. Stories can entertain, educate, and inspire us, while science can reveal the natural world's mysteries and help us understand the Universe we live in. But what happens when these two worlds are integrated? A research review found storytelling a continuous global cultural practice that emphasizes human experiences and conveys wisdom, knowledge, skills, and perspectives.[2] We need science and story to understand the world around us and make it a better place.

2. HEART-CENTERING TECHNIQUES

We've all been there. You have a big decision to make, and your mind is racing. You're trying to think of every outcome and how it will affect you and others. It can feel so overwhelming! To help manage these thoughts and calm the mind, you can use heart-centering techniques.

Heart-centering techniques are internal adjustments designed to help change thoughts and feelings. You come into balance from within, not by using something outside you. Heart-centering can be used in almost any situation in just a few minutes. These techniques involve awareness, intention, imagery, and a grateful heart connection. The process of centering includes taking a moment, breathing deeply, clearing concerns, and consciously gathering your life force energy.[3]

Heart coherence is the harmonious relationship, connection, and correlation in a system.[4] Heart coherence is measurable, using a small sensor and smartphone application. Most of these monitors measure changes in the amount of time between each heartbeat with a finger or earlobe sensor and then provide feedback.[5] If you are interested in monitoring your coherence levels when you apply the heart-centering techniques, search: "biofeedback heart coherence" and select the monitoring device that is right for you. Some of the benefits of heart coherence are stress reduction, health promotion, enhanced creativity, better self-care, emotional regulation, increased intuitive insight, and improved performance.

3. MINDFUL GRATITUDE JOURNAL

We all know that journaling is excellent for self-reflection, discovery, and expression, but what about focusing on being grateful? Recent studies have shown that gratitude has added benefits, such as improved perceived stress levels. Adding gratitude practices into mindful journaling can help us get the most out of both practices.

A research review reported that writing has therapeutic effects for symptoms of distress and promotes psychological well-being![6] Also, another research review described gratitude lists as significantly improving perceived stress and depression.[7] So mindfulness and gratitude go together. The power of gratitude practices and journaling is undeniable. With the right tools, we can choose to go deep with our writing or take a few minutes to focus on being grateful for what we have in life.

4. HEALTHY-HABIT WORKBOOK AND PLANS

We all know that developing healthy habits is key to a happy, successful life. But even when we have the best intentions, it's tough to stay on track day after day. Sticking to healthy habits will help us increase our productivity and well-being. A research review on having a flourishing brain in the twenty-first century described the ten good habits for optimal brain function:

1. Healthy Eating
2. Exercising
3. Rest and Sleep
4. Optimism
5. Managing Stress
6. Making Autonomous Decisions
7. Variety and Challenge
8. Social and Friend Interactions

9. Learning New Things
10. Repetition.[8]

We can achieve optimal well-being by combining self-care, meditation, nutrition, movement, sleep, and healthy emotions. We can continually improve ourselves. Neuroplasticity means we can optimize the connections in our brains for better performance than we currently have.

To make a habit last, it should be: (1) obvious, (2) attractive, (3) easy, and (4) satisfying.[9] Life always poses obstacles, and by using an If-Then Plan we are two to three times more likely to succeed.[10] The Healthy-Habit Check-Ins will help you develop a lifestyle of wellness practices. These habits blend self-reflection and scientific discovery so we can shift from surviving to thriving and flourishing by sticking to our healthy habits.

5. INTENTION AND AFFIRMATION

Intention plays a significant role in how we experience life, especially when it comes to what we can't see with our physical eyes. Just think about all the times you've had an intuition or gut feeling about something before it played out in your life. This book is packed full of affirmations to help you nurture a positive mindset for a life you will love living. Our thoughts and intentions are what create our reality.

GETTING STARTED

Now is our time for well-being and becoming blooming—attractively healthy and full of energy!

It's your road
and yours alone.
Others may walk it
with you, but no one
can walk it for you.

RUMI

**The rose's rarest essence
lives in the thorns.**

RUMI

Aspire & Upgrade
OUR SYSTEMS

If you find the mirror of the heart dull,
the rust has not been cleared from its face. —Rumi

Most people hold a mirror to their living and caring that reflects like a dusty, rusty mirror. In Self-Caring, we learn to polish our mirror's surface to see our inner selves reflected clearly. There are many ways to grow and care for ourselves, but not all come with a book to help us understand ourselves physically, mentally, emotionally, and spiritually. The world can be a harsh place; with perceptions of imperfections in all shapes and sizes, it's easy to forget what makes each of us unique. Even though Self-Caring is part of everyday life, it is not taught in most schools. But don't worry, friend, I have walked this path personally and guided many by my side.

The Self-Caring journey has a tremendous impact.

Most diseases are associated with stress, adversity, or disruption to balance (homeostasis). So getting skilled at surfing the big wave of stress is a much better option than letting it crash down on us. A busy life becomes a happier life when balanced with daily routines and practices that bring peace, mindfulness, gratitude, prosperity, and fulfillment.

Why is there so much negativity in the world?

It is nobody's fault. Negative thoughts take less than a second, while positive thoughts take twelve seconds or more! Human beings are naturally pessimistic and default to using a primitive part of our total system. A research review on negativity bias reported that humans favor negative information more than neutral or positive information.[1] Imagine that, favoring the bad over the good.

It helps when we make a greater effort to use a positive focus.

If we focus on negative things, our default program for life is filled with negativity. On the other hand, if we make a greater effort to focus on positive things, then that is what we will

ASPIRE & UPGRADE OUR SYSTEMS

grow in our lives. I prefer making a greater effort to use a positive focus because like attracts like. If we are mindful, grateful, and focused on positive aspects of any given situation, then the Law of Attraction brings us more of life's positives.

Think back to when computers first came out (if you are too young to have experienced this, search: "image first computer"). They were supersized and slow. If we do not advance our operating systems, our primitive systems prevail. So it makes sense that aspiring to upgrade our systems will bring tremendous benefits.

Envision the first computer again. Now hold up your smartphone. Do you see my point? When smartphones replaced their larger counterparts, they allowed us to live with less gear and save a ton of environmental resources. Now a whole office full of items (scanner, TV, radio, file cabinets, camera, camcorder, calculator, typewriter, tape recorder) fits in your pocket. Some even believe that the smartphone saved the planet (search: "smartphone dematerialization").

Our bodies and minds, the stuff in our homes, offices, cars, and communities all need focus and awareness to stay organized. We can completely reprogram our systems to be more capable and efficient using desire, focus, and attention. This is exciting!

Here are some examples of shifting our looking glass to a more positive view.

SELF-CARING

Before-to-After Negative Thinking Refocusing Techniques:

- ***Before:*** You're tired of feeling that you can't do anything right. You have negative thoughts running through your mind all day long, making you feel bad about yourself.

  After: Imagine being able to choose to see your successes and positive qualities more of the time, so you feel good about yourself and what you do accomplish.

- ***Before:*** You're tired of being stuck in negative and racing thoughts. You've tried to stop yourself from thinking negatively, but it never works for you.

  After: Imagine being able to quickly transform negative thoughts into positives such as appreciation, creating a positive spiral of feeling good.

- ***Before:*** You're tired of being the one who always has a negative outlook on life. You want to be able to look at things positively, but you just can't.

  After: Imagine looking at the world with a cheerful outlook and seeing the good in everything around you. Instead of focusing on what's wrong, you'll notice how beautiful everything is and feel happier.

- ***Before:*** You're tired of being stressed out all the time. Your life is full of anxiety and uncertainty, and you don't know how to manage it.

ASPIRE & UPGRADE OUR SYSTEMS

After: Imagine using a simple technique that helps you reduce anxiety and enhance inner peace.

- *Before:* Life's big stress wave is crashing down on you.

  After: Image surfing the big stress wave in a natural flow with the ocean.

As we learn to pay attention to our inner selves and where we're going on our journeys, we will access our highest and best well-being, self-growth, and caring potentials. This book is a safe space for us to explore and learn practices to help us rebalance, grow, and flow through life with greater *ease* and *wellness* (the opposites of *dis-ease* and *illness*).

Once we grow our inner resources, we awaken our highest and best abilities. Then we explore more about the history of caring to strengthen our roots. When we have deep, strong roots, it will be much harder for life's challenges to push us down. As our Self-Caring abilities expand and grow, we say goodbye to self-doubt and guilt, create vibrant health, boost mental clarity, deepen creativity, and improve relationships.

Welcome to our Self-Caring Revival, friend. It's time to discover, activate, grow, and nurture our highest and best well-being, self-growth, and caring potential. We have a deep, natural desire to care for ourselves. I know it's difficult sometimes, but we are always worth the effort! We can upgrade and

SELF-CARING

redesign our systems to feel more energized, creative, socially connected, and spiritually grounded.

This chapter has given some tips on cultivating our inner genius and how to start strengthening our roots. I hope each of us takes what resonates with us today and starts putting it into practice in small ways. As our caring practices grow stronger with time, they will soon become second nature. Our lives are too precious not to prioritize taking care of ourselves.

PERSONAL POWER POINTS

1. *We must focus harder on seeing the positives.*
2. *What we choose to focus on is what we grow.*
3. *Our integrated system (mind-body-soul) nurtures our highest and best well-being, self-growth, and caring potentials.*

MEET
Our Guide

I will soothe you and heal you. I will bring you roses.
I too, have been covered with thorns. —Rumi

Along my Self-Caring journey, I met someone capable of teaching me how to fuel up from the inside. His messages are still undeniably the most thought-provoking I have ever pondered. At times his words crack my heart open, bring me to tears, and soothe me all at the same time. In a noble and great city, his story goes back to the thirteenth century.

In Balkh, an ancient city in what is today northern Afghanistan, a leading scholar and theologian, Baha al-Din, was forced to leave his home. A group of disciples, his family, and his five-year-old boy, Jalaluddin, traveled with him as they set out westward. When they passed through the city of Nishapur, they met Fariduddin Attar, a celebrated Persian poet. Attar immediately recognized the young boy's spiritual eminence. He presented the boy with a *Book of Mysteries* (about the soul and the material world) and foretold that he would someday become famous.

The travelers settled in Iconium, an ancient Roman province. This became their home, and here the boy was called Rumi (the Roman). During his last years, Rumi composed the *Masnavi*, a six-volume poem with metaphysics, fables, scenes, interpretations, and revelations about living.[1]

Rumi is one of the greatest interpreters of wholeness.

Rumi is a beautiful rose in the garden of spirit. He represents "being blooming," and he can easily guide us on our journey. Rumi knows how to live mindfully and how we can reach our highest and best well-being, self-growth, and caring potential. Our journey will be more meaningful as we consider his messages.

Rumi's focus is unique and may feel foreign at first, but he is just like us in many ways. Rumi learned from his mistakes in life, which allowed him to help others. He knows that every-one makes mistakes and falters along the way. But he

MEET OUR GUIDE

also knows how to love life and how to celebrate life. Rumi can teach us a lot about focusing on seeing our experiences as beautiful in some way, even the painful ones.

We can learn a lot from Rumi about caring for ourselves and the world around us. It's not good to depend on others for our happiness, especially if their suffering is more significant than ours.

We also don't want to be a prisoner of our past—locked up and stuck. Nor a victim of a future of worry. Rumi guides us to live in the present moment because this way of living sets us free and allows us to create our desired futures.

The gift of living in the present moment frees us from memories that keep us stuck and from future worries.

Rumi knew that everyone slips up occasionally. Yet he wanted the best for everyone, and his timeless words of wisdom can help us today to find ways to exist in prosperity, peace, and joy, as he did. Rumi, like everyone else, struggled with darkness. But despite these obstacles, he found ways to exist in prosperity.

Rumi's poetic messages will help us feel supported, safe, and stable along our journey. Rumi will also help us rise above dark moments, but he cannot do it for us. So it is best to put

SELF-CARING

in the effort and keep growing and moving forward on our path. We are strong enough to overcome obstacles along the way, knowing that these problems help make us stronger. The more challenging something seems, the greater the chance for growth. I hope that when we receive a message from Rumi, we feel safe and supported on our journey.

Whoever travels without a guide, needs two hundred years for a two-day journey. —*Rumi*

PERSONAL POWER POINTS

1. Living in the present moment sets us free.
2. Bringing awareness to negative emotions activates our power of conscious choice to change them in the present moment.
3. Seeking the growth potential in each obstacle turns our wounds into wisdom.

**The wound is
the place where the light
enters you.**

RUMI

MINDFUL GRATITUDE JOURNAL

STEP 1
Aspire

AFFIRMATION:

I commit to growing my potential.

Pause after each question. Answer by asking, "What is most on my heart today?"

How do I feel about my well-being, self-growth, and caring journey?

SELF-CARING

Do I have hope and optimism, or other feelings?

What are some skills and talents that to me feel like fun but to others feel like work?

What activities make me lose track of time?

What comes naturally to me in life, relationships, or work?

What are aspects of my personality or body that I don't like?

If I am talking to my best friend, how would I rewrite what I just beat myself up for?

SELF-CARING

What will I commit to doing each day to connect with myself positively?

1.

2.

3.

4.

5.

6.

7.

Example: I will commit each day to place my hand on my heart and offer gratitude to my heart for watching over me.

MINDFUL GRATITUDE JOURNAL · STEP 1: ASPIRE

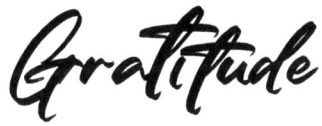

Gratitude makes my heart sing.

What three people or pets do I feel grateful for having in my life?

1.

2.

3.

What three items do I feel grateful for having in my life?

1.

2.

3.

SELF-CARING

What can I do to be more kind to myself?

1.

2.

3.

4.

5.

6.

7.

Example: I will replace negative thoughts with positive ones.

You were born with potential. You were born with goodness and trust. You were born with ideals and dreams. You were born with greatness. You have wings. Learn to use them and fly.

RUMI

HEALTHY-HABIT WORKBOOK

STEP 1
Aspire

AFFIRMATION:

My lifelong journey takes me to all the places where I need to grow.

THE TECHNIQUE OF HEART-CENTERING

Now, let's continue to focus on connecting with our inner selves by using a mindfulness technique I call heart-centering. Focused awareness (mindfulness in the present moment) on negative thoughts can prevent them from escalating out of control.[2] By not suppressing our emotions, we gain the power of conscious choice to change them in the present moment.

My favorite way to fully appreciate and come into the present moment is to use a heart-centering technique to activate my inner genius. Heart-centering can take us out of reactivity or negativity into a more conscious state, where we can choose a more soothing response. The wonderful thing about using heart-centering is that it also improves many of our natural abilities, like deepening creativity and improving health, as we learn to live in coherence, which is the opposite of disorder. I often refer to coherence as flow.

I center myself before teaching, writing, creating, and every time somebody frustrates me. I can get back into flow about 90 percent of the time using a few minutes of heart-centering. The 10 percent of the time I continue to escalate, I slip away and lock myself in the bathroom until I calm down. My favorite saying is, "It is better to run away than to have to pay."

Everyone has troubled times. Just like the rose, we all have thorns. Gratitude opens self-awareness, while fear, anger, and resentment block awareness. Gently calming your breathing and focusing on your heart of creation in your upper chest expands self-awareness.

HEART-CENTERING

Begin by breathing in and out slowly and deeply three times. You can use a count of five as you breathe in and five as you breathe out. Of course, a comfortable breathing pace is the most important, so if you need to slow or speed up your breath, this is perfectly fine. Feel the ground beneath you as our planet holds you safely.

Imagine your breath flowing in and out of your upper chest area as you continue to breathe. Allow your breath to flow in and out smoothly, slowly, and deeply.

Now imagine your upper chest is a beautiful flower. Breathe in the beauty of your flower. Continue to breathe slowly and deeply, allowing your breath to flow in and out of your fragrant petals.

Breathe in gratitude for the beauty of your flower.

Allow gratitude to fill up your heart.

Now continue to breathe in a way that feels comfortable.

HEALTHY-HABIT CHECK-IN

Select three habits to focus on this week.

1. Healthy Eating

This week I will eat a healthy, balanced diet. The food on my plate will be colorful like a rainbow.

2. Exercising

I will move my body to get my heart pumping at least three times this week (like running, biking, yoga, dancing, hiking, or nature walking solo or with a friend).

3. Variety and Challenge

This week I will do something out of my usual routine (like try a different type of activity, sign up for a new program, or eat at a new place).

4. Learning New Things

I will spend time this week on one new active form of leisure (like volunteering or studying a new language or form of creative expression).

5. Managing Stress

When I am waiting for someone this week, I will embrace the opportunity to take several deep and slow mindful breaths, feeling how good it is to inhale and exhale fully.

INTENTIONS

INTENTION:

Whenever
(situation arises), I will respond by

I can ask for anything. What am I asking the Universe for?

OPTIMIZING PLAN:

I will do
for this amount of time:
in this place:
starting **and**
repeating every

IF-THEN PLAN:

If
then I will remain flexible and instead

I once needed
other people and
items to validate my worth,
but this felt like pushing a giant
boulder up a steep mountain. I was
moving in the wrong direction by
trying to repair the broken. I bloomed
when I learned to nurture myself
using my inner wholeness.
Now I live in flow, and I can
jump over mountains.

MICHELLE PECK

· PART II ·
Belonging

Your task is not to seek for Love but merely
to seek and find all the barriers within yourself that
you have built against it.

RUMI

The whole Universe
is contained within a
single Human Being, You.

RUMI

UNLOCK THE
Door of Belonging

How can we find more peace within ourselves?

There was a time when my surroundings were unpredictable. My childhood home ranged from nurturing to ice-cold to reactive rage. As a result, I lived in discomfort from the anticipation of not knowing what was coming next. I learned to always be on guard, so much so that my neck often was stiff, painful, and would lock in a fixed position. In the fifth-grade science fair, I wore a red-checkered dress and explained the scientific method with my head frozen tilted to the left with an intoxicating scent of peppermint coming from the cream layered on my neck. I looked and smelled like a candy cane and kept praying that the

SELF-CARING

judges liked peppermint while trying desperately to straighten my head.

In 1999 I was a young college student at the University of Texas at El Paso. In one class the student next to me sat there bragging about his acceptance to a school in Houston. All I could think was, *well, if he can go to school in Houston, I can too.* So later that afternoon, I walked to the basement chemistry lab to use the computer. A few searches and several hours later, I had completed my application for a nursing program in Houston.

In the scorching summer of 2000, my family packed all my belongings into our seven-seater van, and I followed them 800-plus miles to Houston. The van's air-conditioning broke about midway, and my sister turned red, drenched in sweat. We reached Houston, picked up some supplies, and then I was alone in my one-bedroom apartment. My mind became quiet after I turned on the radio and relaxed. Everything from this day forward was now only up to me.

The Texas Medical Center (the largest medical center in the world) was like nothing I had ever seen before. Many times, I felt as if Houston were swallowing me up—especially during my first year of nursing school, when Tropical Storm Allison left me without access to school for weeks due to disaster and flooding. But despite all the craziness, I was filled with gratitude for this opportunity to improve my life. Each time I waited at the bus stop, soaked in sweat from the scorching Houston heat, I smiled in deep gratitude. I was reinventing my life.

As a new nurse, I needed to stay busy. After working and attending classes Monday through Friday, I would work two twelve-hour shifts in the hospital on the weekends. I felt this urgent need to stay busy because:

1. It helped me calm my racing mind.
2. I was climbing a steep career-building mountain.
3. I sought attention, affection, acceptance, and appreciation.

Many years later, in 2009, after a few years of running my first company as a nurse practitioner, the phone rang, and my mother's voice was on the other end of the line. I explained all about my business successes and profits. My mother simply replied that she was happy for me. But she did not tell me the affirmation I needed to hear. I felt disappointed. She passed the phone to my father. I again explained my career triumphs, and he too simply replied he was happy for me. I needed more. As I hung up the phone, I fell to my knees, and I begged for a better way.

Why was I still hurting despite now having full approval from my parents?

SELF-CARING

I waited for my answer to come, and a few weeks later, it arrived. As I turned on the television, a local pastor appeared on the screen with tears in his eyes, preaching that we are all born with crowns on our heads. I realized that I had complete control over my kingdom. At this moment, I felt different about myself. I felt uplifted and hopeful. I had a new focus for my looking glass. I decided to focus my life on learning to reconnect to my wholeness from that day forward.

> **Inside any deep asking is the answering.**
> RUMI

This new focus awakened my sense of belonging; I discovered my inner genius. I realized that I was already whole and not broken. I was not a sum of parts. Externalizing self-worth by placing value on other people's decisions, feelings, and actions is a recipe for disappointment.

> **Why are you so enchanted by this world when a mine of gold lies within you?**
> RUMI

I also learned that the Universe is a reliable source of information. Trust and allow your answers to unfold. I also discovered that holding my parents responsible for my sense of belonging kept me locked in survival mode, powerless, and suffering. My self-worth was not something that I could earn or place on others.

UNLOCK THE DOOR OF BELONGING

Learning that I was worthy even before I was born opened my awareness—I came here from the highest source of energy: Love. And this is me. I belonged to Love even before I got to Earth, and I will belong to Love for eternity (even after my human body ceases to be). This focus allowed grace to begin flowing in my everyday living.

We all can immerse back into our inner genius. This choice is available at any given moment. Imagine the world as a canvas, the body the paint, and the inner genius the artist.

Don't let memories use and confuse; let go and move forward. We are much more than we could ever imagine.

As soon as we are born, thoughts start manifesting in unique ways. As we learn to care for ourselves from our inner selves, we will experience a profound difference. Living our highest and best Self-Caring begins with belonging.

When we are young, there is always a struggle to fit in. Surroundings like schools, social networks, and even our families can become places where we try to please others. Unfortunately, pleasing others, often to survive, takes precedence over living from our inner selves. Needing to be heard, seen, and valued leads to seeking approval and pleasing others outside ourselves. Clearing the dust off our mirrors is the most crucial step.

SELF-CARING

Now, after more than twenty years in nursing, I know that it was gratitude that salvaged me from the scorching heat at the Houston bus stop. But it wasn't until I unlocked the door to belonging that my healing activated.

We are so much more than what happened yesterday or even this morning. Our future is still unwritten because it's up to us how we live today. Open to new possibilities by living with an open heart full of gratitude, and grace will flow! Let's continue to focus on connecting with our inner selves and optimizing self-caring.

PERSONAL POWER POINTS

1. *We are already whole, not broken, and worthy even before we were born.*
2. *We belong for eternity to Infinite Love.*
3. *Unlocking the door to belonging is crucial for cultivating our well-being.*

You think of
yourself as a citizen
of the Universe. You think
you belong to this world of
dust and matter. Out of this
dust, you have created a
personal image and have
forgotten about the essence
of your true origin.

RUMI

MINDFUL GRATITUDE JOURNAL

STEP 2
Wholeness

AFFIRMATION:

My highest and best potential activates when I embrace body, mind, heart, soul, and spirit.

Pause after each question. Answer by asking, "What is most on my heart today?"

How have my thorns grown me?

SELF-CARING

How does accepting myself, even with imperfections, help my relationships?

What qualities and talents do I need to have recognized by a coworker, family member, or friend?

What skills have I developed because of challenges?

MINDFUL GRATITUDE JOURNAL · STEP 2: WHOLENESS

What fears are am I interested in transforming?

Gratitude

To help me look at the sunny side up of life, I'll describe three bright things, pets, or people that shine in my life.

1 ·

2 ·

3 ·

HEALTHY-HABIT WORKBOOK

STEP 2
Wholeness

AFFIRMATION:

**I begin with belonging
and live my authentic truth.**

HEART-CENTERING

Begin by breathing in and out slowly and deeply three times. You can use a count of five as you breathe in and five as you breathe out; this is a good slow and steady pace. Now continue to breathe at whatever rate feels comfortable to you and whisper these words quietly inside to yourself:

"I am much more than I believe."
"I am a unique expression of energy."
"I am a masterpiece in progress."

SELF-CARING

"I exist, belong, and always have."

"I live and grow with purpose."

"I connect to my life and others."

"Creation celebrates me."

"I have tremendous worth and value."

"I continue to grow freely in the gift the present moment gives me."

Now continue to breathe in a way that feels comfortable.

> **Heart-centering shifts chaos to coherence, aligning with wholeness and healing.**
>
> MICHELLE PECK

HEALTHY-HABIT CHECK-IN

Select three habits to focus on this week.

1. Healthy Eating

This week, I will buy a piece of food that I love. I will savor it with all five senses and enjoy it for at least ten minutes.

2. Exercising

I will walk in nature and notice as many details as I can as I pass by. What color are the leaves? What types of trees and wildlife did I see? What is in bloom? What is in the sky?

3. Rest and Sleep

Caffeine and blue light mess up my sleep. This week, I will reduce electronic use two hours before bed and not consume caffeinated food or drinks after mid-morning.

4. Making Autonomous Decisions

This week, I will turn a mundane act like being stuck in traffic into an enjoyable action like listening to an audiobook while waiting.

5. Social and Friend Interactions

Social interactions make my brain better. This week, I will focus on creating positive social relationships to promote my health and well-being.

SELF-CARING

INTENTIONS

INTENTION:

Whenever _____
(situation arises), I will respond by _____
_____

I can ask for anything. What am I asking the Universe for?
_____
_____

OPTIMIZING PLAN:

I will do _____
for this amount of time: _____
in this place: _____
starting _____ **and**
repeating every _____

IF-THEN PLAN:

If _____
then I will remain flexible and instead _____
_____

STEP THROUGH THE
Doorway of Belonging

> Grace is the door to the
> peace beyond the mind. —Rumi

*I*n 2018 I was sitting in the back of the room. Two colleagues stood up and asked for volunteer facilitators, and I offered my help.

Then something happened that changed my life forever.

I showed up for the first session, and I looked down at the sign-in sheet. My heart drummed against my chest, and I felt paralyzed by fear. I was a participant in all the sessions, not a facilitator. I took a deep, cleansing breath and considered all the benefits of participating versus facilitating. Going to happy hour with my peers came to mind. Yep, that was it. Of course, the main advantage is that you can go to happy hour with your fellow participants.

I called up my courage and signed in. Boxes of crayons and stacks of pastel paper sat on the table. I took a small box of crayons and a sheet of yellow paper and sat in the back of the room.

The real facilitator guided us in a mindful breathing practice and then instructed us to draw the part we leave at home every day. I panicked and scanned the room for other non-drawers, but everyone was coloring on their papers. So I started daydreaming about happy hour, picked up a black crayon, and began sketching my hidden self.

Within a few minutes, I had filled the entire paper. I quickly tucked my drawing into my folder to keep it safe and hidden away. Then the facilitator explained—we would now go to smaller rooms to share our drawings with the other participants. My problem-solving brain kicked in immediately as I slumped down in my chair, scanned the room, and started crafting a getaway plan. I would quietly slip away during the room transition, not come back, and meet my best friend at happy hour to debrief about the horror. A stellar plan.

Within seconds I started along my escape path, but some fellow participants caught up to me. They expressed excitement about being in the same group with me. Ugh! My stellar plan had failed, so I lied, "I'm so happy to be in a group with you too." Then I told the truth, "But I'm not the facilitator. I'm a participant like you." All our eyes got big as we held the look of disbelief. They had only known me as Professor Peck.

Six of us sat down and introduced ourselves to the group. Everyone looked at me with disbelief when I gulped and introduced myself as Michelle. Then the facilitator asked us to place our drawing on the floor in the center of our circled chairs. I was terrified and almost passed out as my thoughts started racing.

I sneaked a peek at the student to my left, who calmly placed the drawing down in the middle of the circle. They all placed their pictures in the middle—casually! I reluctantly opened my folder, clutched my drawing with trembling hands, and tried my best to release it gently into the center of the circle.

We took turns disclosing our hidden selves by describing our drawings. I tried desperately not to cry, but tears spilled from my eyes.

Then something incredible happened.

As I listened deeply to each story, a warmth filled my body, my mind calmed, and I felt at peace. Everybody was leaving pieces of themselves at home. It wasn't just me.

SELF-CARING

When it was my turn, I considered passing, but instead, I called up my courage and described my drawing. A black framed mirror covered the right half of the paper, filled with red and pink hearts of all shapes and sizes. Two enormous green eyes covered the left half of the page. They were gazing into the mirror. These eyes were mine. And the words "UNIVERSAL LOVE" arched over the top of the page.

> **As you start to walk on the way, the way appears.**
>
> RUMI

As tears spilled from my eyes, I explained that during my life, learning about the soul came from those I read, watched, and listened to at home. I kept this part of me separate from my teaching at the university. Rumi and my spiritual teachers did not pass through the university doorway.

But during my clinical geriatric nursing practice, I had learned long ago that a person became a heaping mess without mind-body-soul integration. The only way to make sense of the typical client visit (ten medications, diagnoses, and specialists) was to hold them in wholeness. So I began seeing new clients and viewing them as you would a whole meal rather than focusing on each separate ingredient—which is honestly an impossible task in a forty-five-minute visit. Heaps of ingredients forced me long ago to learn how to step away from the parts and focus on wholeness, the only way to support recovery and healing.

STEP THROUGH THE DOORWAY OF BELONGING

As tears flowed down my face, I realigned with my hidden self and embraced all of myself back into wholeness. This was the undeniable power of the peer-support group (also called a healing circle). My life forever changed.

I learned how to speak up from my inner self. The safety and comfort of the peer-support group allowed me to experience belonging in a place where I had separated from my inner self to fit in.

> **Be like a tree and let the dead leaves drop.**
>
> RUMI

I took a vow that day. I would never separate mind-body-soul again, no matter what. I accepted myself entirely and have walked through every doorway, including the university, in my wholeness from that day forward. My teaching abilities, well-being, self-growth, and caring skyrocketed because of this one vow.

The peer group healing circle created a safe space that helped me walk through the doorway of belonging. I cleaned the dust off my mirror's surface, and next, I would learn to polish my mirror.

Do you ever feel that you're always trying to please someone other than yourself?

SELF-CARING

Everyone has problems, fears, and pains. But unfortunately, we are so eager to do the work of healing ourselves physically within our comfort zones that we neglect what is the most challenging, and rewarding, aspect—healing ourselves emotionally and spiritually. Unfortunately, we suffer just as much from emotional and spiritual wounds as physical ones; they are only more hidden. And often, our emotional scars feel like a burden rather than an asset to nurture.

I have felt rejected on countless occasions.

We all need to belong, to have a tribe that accepts us wholly and does not see us as a bunch of broken pieces. During childhood, I learned to silence my inner voice in my family to better fit in, and I carried this into my career.

Although I continue to walk in my wholeness with my authentic voice, there are challenges. The hardest part is setting boundaries, like knowing when to stand up or stay silent. Some days, I have significant challenges, depending on those surrounding me. But other days, when surrounded by my peer group healing circle enthusiasts, I sit in grace.

I know the struggles of needing to be accepted.

STEP THROUGH THE DOORWAY OF BELONGING

Our path to embracing belonging is the worthiest challenge thinkable. It takes courage to open self-awareness. The artistry is in reaching beyond simply wanting to belong. It takes great courage to live your light and beam it to connect with all that surrounds you.

Our journey is much easier when we are surrounded by supporters.

Some of us are born with a natural ability to relate. We know how to make friends, feel safe in groups, and be comfortable talking about our feelings or vulnerabilities no matter the situation. But for many of us, this is not the case. It's tough when we don't have an innate sense of belonging because it can make us feel alone in life—without a defined purpose and connection. If this sounds familiar, then the path takes time, but each step is worth every ounce of effort.

We may need some help opening new doors to gain more self-awareness, grow courage, trust, and finally, understand all aspects of who we are. Professional counselors and peer support groups like those at Healing Circles Global are excellent ways to support our journey.

SELF-CARING

PERSONAL POWER POINTS

1 · *Our scars (thorns) are assets to nurture.*
2 · *Once we walk through the doorway of belonging, we take a vow never to turn back.*
3 · *Well-being, self-growth, and caring are more manageable around supporters.*

Eternal life glitters
on the leaves of the garden.
The flowers will blaze,
and the bird cries shower us
with immortality.

RUMI

Belonging MANIFESTO

Whenever I am unsure of what to do or say, especially around non-supporters, I activate one aspect of my Belonging Manifesto to guide me. This way, I reside in my wholeness while keeping good boundaries.

ASPECT ONE

The art of knowing is knowing what to ignore. Ignore those that make you fearful and sad, that degrade you back towards disease and death. —*Rumi*

ASPECT TWO

When unsure of what to say or do, first choose silence. If necessary, excuse yourself politely—I need to use the restroom, let me get back to you on that—then rest and reflect. In silence and contemplation, ask for clarity. —*Michelle Peck*

ASPECT THREE

Always search for your innermost nature in those you are with, as rose oil imbibes from roses. —*Rumi*

ASPECT FOUR

People can only act from their level of self-awareness. It's not your job to fix, judge, or change anyone. Give these jobs back to the Universe. —*Michelle Peck*

ASPECT FIVE

By focusing on your personal growth, each moment becomes a new opportunity for offering kindness to yourself. —*Michelle Peck*

ASPECT SIX

I belong to the beloved, have seen the two worlds as one and that one call to and know. First, last, outer, inner, only that breath breathing, human being. —*Rumi*

ASPECT SEVEN

The very center of your heart is where life begins. The most beautiful place on Earth. —*Rumi*

MINDFUL GRATITUDE JOURNAL

STEP 3
Courage

AFFIRMATION:

**I always have a choice
when I open my mind and heart.**

*Pause after each question. Answer by asking,
"What is most on my heart today?"*

Describe the benefits of walking through the doorway of belonging.

_____
_____
_____
_____

SELF-CARING

What does belonging mean?

Who are my greatest allies?

Describe these relationships.

What am I learning from those who oppose me?

Describe these relationships.

SELF-CARING

My Belonging
MANIFESTO

My Belonging Manifesto guides my boundaries.

ASPECT ONE

_____
_____
_____
_____
_____

ASPECT TWO

_____
_____
_____
_____
_____

ASPECT THREE

ASPECT FOUR

ASPECT FIVE

Gratitude

Write about an event (something that happened) during the past few weeks that left me feeling satisfied.

How did this event help me achieve this feeling of satisfaction?

Light and dark coexist.
Dark cannot dim your light.
The load you bear weighs you
down. Unpack your bags
to beam your light.

MICHELLE PECK

HEALTHY-HABIT WORKBOOK

STEP 3
Courage

AFFIRMATION:

I am curious, creative, and commit to lifelong learning.

HEART-CENTERING

Begin by breathing in and out slowly and deeply three times. You can use a count of five as you breathe in and five as you breathe out; this is a good slow and steady pace. Continue breathing comfortably and imagine a tightly closed flower bud in your upper chest area. The flower wants to peek out, but nature has not allowed for this quite yet. Nurture the flower with your breath. Breathe slowly and deeply into your upper chest as you focus on nurturing the flower with your breath.

SELF-CARING

At the right moment, the bloom will open and unfold its petaled beauty. But if the flower pushes and opens too early, its ultimate potential gets limited, and the bloom will never be as magnificent and fragrant as it would become by growing in ease and flowing with nature.

As you breathe into the flower, it unfolds gently on the out-breath in perfect alignment with nature.

Now continue to breathe in a way that feels comfortable.

> **Activating the courage to live our authentic truths is healing.**
>
> MICHELLE PECK

HEALTHY-HABIT CHECK-IN

Select three habits to focus on this week.

1. Healthy Eating

This week, I will eat slow carbs (like vegetables, whole grains, and legumes) because they give a steady supply of energy to my body and brain, unlike fast carbs in sweets.

2. Exercising

This week, I will have a mindful hike on a nature path and notice nature's beauty as I pass by.

3. Rest and Sleep

Sleep helps my brain and emotional skills. Without enough, learning suffers, and toxins are stored in my body. This week I will get sufficient sleep, seven hours for most adults.

4. Optimism

My cells are listening to my thoughts, so I will nurture my cells by thinking positive thoughts this week. I will also give attention to my self-talk to boost self-esteem.

5. Social and Friend Interactions

Positive social interactions promote good health and well-being. This week I will be mindful about creating positive social encounters.

INTENTIONS

INTENTION:

Whenever _____
(situation arises), I will respond by _____
_____

I can ask for anything. What am I asking the Universe for?
_____
_____

OPTIMIZING PLAN:

I will do _____
for this amount of time: _____
in this place: _____
starting _____ **and**
repeating every _____

IF-THEN PLAN:

If _____
then I will remain flexible and instead _____
_____

Belonging Before
BEING, KNOWING & DOING

*Knowing takes you to the threshold
but not to the door.* —Rumi

As a teenager in the hot desert of El Paso, Texas, I learned a great deal during lunchtime. I grew up loving Mexican food, and my mother could easily convince me to join her on lunch dates at our favorite restaurants. But, across the table filled with tortilla soup, enchiladas, tacos, and warm chips with fresh salsa, my mother would vent her frustrations and resentments to me. As a result, I became a teenage pseudo-counselor.

My mother did not have a support system as she believed that seeing a professional counselor was a weakness. Her goal was to hold the family together, and she felt that she was stronger

SELF-CARING

by not seeking professional advice. Despite trying hundreds of times, I never could convince her to talk to a professional. As I listened, meal after meal, year after year, trying to fix my mother, my stomach filled with delicious food, but my heart filled with resentment.

> **The moment you accept what troubles you've been given, the door will open.**
>
> RUMI

As a teenage pseudo-counselor, I learned the hard way that books were my best friends. My mother was a reading teacher, so she took me to the bookstore all the time. My pseudo-counselor job brought many responsibilities, guilts, and frustrations. But one day at the bookstore, I found a life-changing book: *Love, Medicine & Miracles* by Bernie Siegal.

As a teenager I tried so hard to fix my mother's problems. But this one book helped me change the focus of my looking glass to view the lunch sessions as lessons preparing me for my future. And I realized that everybody is on a path needed for them to grow. By learning to hold onto less resentment, I began to feel lighter, less burdened, and more comfortable. I learned to listen without needing to fix. Embracing a self-growth perspective began transforming my life and upgrading my system.

I fully upgraded my system and transformed my life using Caring Science.

BELONGING *BEFORE* BEING, KNOWING & DOING

Caring Science is a human scientific discipline that starts with existence.[1] Everything begins with belonging (see Figure 1). Embracing and knowing that you belong to the source of Infinite Love must come before being, becoming, knowing, and doing. Unfortunately, knowing and doing are the most prized and awarded commodities in health, wellness, caring, and healing, and many have missed the most crucial first step.

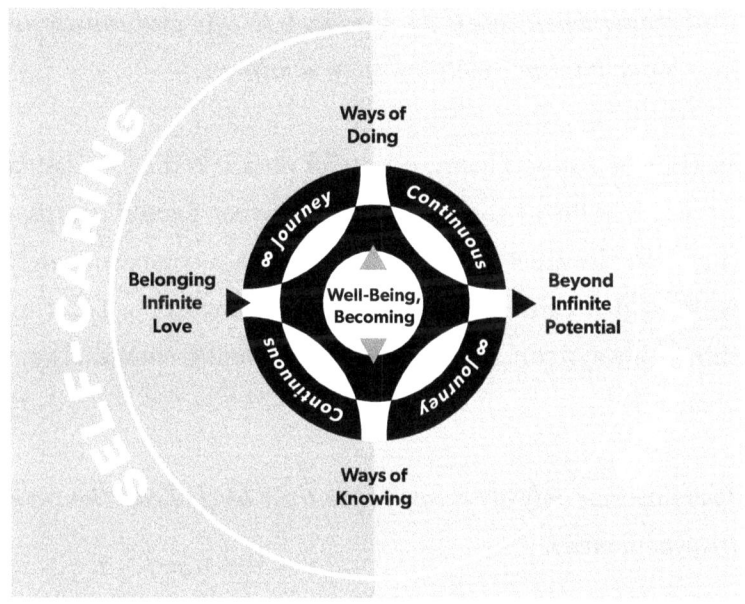

Figure 1. Academy of Well-Being Framework

In Caring Science, we belong even before we are born. We come from source energy of the highest frequency, Infinite Love. Embracing Infinite Love, instead of searching for approval, allows your energy to flow with nature. This harmony brings healing to your heart, mind, body, and the Universe. The caring journey leads you to remember that you belong to Infinite Love.

We are all interconnected. We are whole, complete, and we recognize this when we embrace belonging. While on Earth, we can choose to work with our thinking mind to gain awareness in our inner wisdom center.

Embracing wholeness is an approach to life, and consciousness is our internal relationship to wholeness.

In Human Caring Theory, caring for oneself is the foundation we must build to sustain caring for other people compassionately.[2] In other words, you cannot care compassionately without first caring for oneself fully. Therefore, Self-Caring should always come first, just like belonging should always come first.

Everyone can only act according to their level of consciousness (self-awareness).

By expanding our awareness, we increase our choices. In the *Map of Consciousness,* you move from surviving to thriving at the level of courage.[3] Courage is where you find the door of belonging. "I" begins shifting to "We," and what was once an individual-survivalist-illness focus expands to a group-collective-wellness focus. The collective "We" power, when in coherence, shines like a laser beam, whereas the personal "I" power shines like a light bulb. Therefore, surrounding yourself with professionals and support groups that are in coherence can be more potent for healing than working through something alone.

Caring is a supreme life force that is the foundation of grace, mercy, and the deep source of authentic living, knowing, birthing, and dying.[4] Once we establish our inner genius, we can better perform the ways of being and becoming to access more ways of knowing and doing. These renewed interactions between being and doing lead to renewed ways of living.[5] Finally, shifting from Self-Caring into We-Caring (caring with others) expands human knowledge, behaviors, and understanding. In essence, nurturing a self-reflective practice with a focus on the ways of being and becoming, not only raises personal coherence, but can co-create coherence in people around us (the collective).

Healing activates once we awaken and embrace belonging. Cures and treatments won't always reach the root causes of symptoms, but Infinite Love will. The twenty-first century is a time when the world can now be viewed as a complete system, interacting together. And in this system, all things are natural elements in an entire whole.[6]

***

What is the nature of knowing?

SELF-CARING

When the mind comes into a concentrated state in the present moment, it becomes a mirror that opens to all ways of knowing, moving beyond the mind and measurement. From the caring-healing modalities to healing arts, space opens for shared humanity, humanizing care, and revitalizing health. Self-awareness promotes a higher knowledge of intuition or inner knowing. When we allow our inner knowing, we fully connect.

The amount of new knowledge generated daily is impossible to learn and is outdated rapidly (search terms: "knowledge doubling," "truth decay," and "half-life of facts"). Thankfully, advances in technology and artificial intelligence can help make sense of the massive amounts of knowledge. But where does this leave human beings? With a great need to upgrade our systems.

All this becomes more manageable by viewing symptoms as messengers of disconnection (illness) or of connection (wellness). The underlying emotions and beliefs of disconnection cause physical and emotional disconnections in our bodies. They include feelings like fear, anger, hopelessness, resentment, inadequacy, blaming, and pushing away what's sustaining. But by focusing on connection, body-mind-soul integration, or wholeness rather than parts, symptoms dissipate, and we feel lighter, calmer, and more at peace.

Many experiences shape our lives. When something terrible happens in our life, it can be easy to get lost in that event or series of events. But there is always some glimmer of a positive aspect in everything. When something terrible happens, there is the opportunity to explore what we have learned from the ordeal. One of the most significant ways to open awareness is learning the artistry of forgiveness.

> **These pains you feel are messengers. Listen to them.**
>
> RUMI

We are not alone. I have been there too, and we grow our fullness by getting back to belonging with time and dedication. Let's take a deep breath now, and exhale as you focus on all the things that make up who we are today—our experiences, both good and bad, that shape our lives. There is the power to heal wounds by learning to embrace our inner selves again.

PERSONAL POWER POINTS

1. *Continue to nurture and expand well-being, self-growth, and caring.*
2. *Symptoms are messengers of imbalance. Listen to them.*
3. *After we embrace our inner genius, we can expand the ways of being and becoming to access more ways of knowing and doing.*

Here are some notes with examples of the ways of belonging-being-becoming-knowing-doing. These are the most common ones I have come across along my journey; there are always more . . . much more.

BELONGING

Cosmos, Cosmic Love

Infinite, Universal Love

Wholeness, Oneness, Grace

Infinity of Human Spirit

Unity Consciousness

The Face, Belonging Before Being by Lévinas'

Holding Other in Our Hands by Longstrup

Caring Ethic of Belonging

The Glance by Rumi

Authenticity

Essential Nature

Inner, True, Higher, Highest, Authentic Self

**WAYS OF BEING
& BECOMING**

Caritas-Veritas Light on Virtues

Evolution of Consciousness

Compassion

Forgiveness

Surrender

Resiliency

Metaphysical

Focus of Mind

Energy Field

Frequency Wave Resonance

WAYS OF DOING

Skills, Tasks

Lifestyle Practices

Procedures

Interventions

Techniques, Tools

Modalities, Rituals

Research, Praxis

WAYS OF KNOWING

Laws, Rules, Theories

Universal Principles

Qualitative

Quantitative

Empirical

Ethical

Political

Personal

Lived Experience

Facts

Aesthetics

Patterns

Unknowing

Cultural

Intuitive, Innate

Mythologic

Archetypes

Access your
inner self using the
in-and-out breath and
embrace self-kindness. Each time
self-rejection and judgment cloud
your mirror's surface, gently wipe
the dust away. Continue to
polish your mirror with
gratitude and Self-Caring.

MICHELLE PECK

MINDFUL GRATITUDE JOURNAL

STEP 4
Belonging

AFFIRMATION:

I choose how I see, hear, and value myself.

Emotions are experienced in two ways: comfort or discomfort.

1. *Comfort*—move us from constriction (feeling tight) to expansion (feeling free).
2. *Discomfort*—constrict us (feeling tight, pains), keeping us stuck.

Pause after each question. Answer by asking, "What is most on my heart today?"

SELF-CARING

My most common comforting, freeing, and unstuck feelings are:

1.
2.
3.

My most common discomforting, tight, painful, or stuck feelings are:

1.
2.
3.

Three of my most common symptoms are . . . and my needs that are not being met when I experience these symptoms are:

1.

2.

3.

MINDFUL GRATITUDE JOURNAL · STEP 4: BELONGING

As I am growing my connections and experiences, I would like to grow more:

What can I let go of to help myself grow?

SELF-CARING

What am I growing in these seven focus areas?

1. Physical Body and Mental Wellness

---

2. Spiritual and Emotional Wellness

---

3. Family and Friends

---

4. Career, Leisure, and Hobbies

---

5. Public Service

---

6. Self-Caring Practices

---

7. Material Possessions

MY 5-STEP PLAN THAT NOURISHES MY BELONGING

STEP 1

STEP 2

STEP 3

STEP 4

STEP 5

SELF-CARING

Gratitude

My favorite activities that make me happy are:

1.

2.

3.

4.

5.

6.

7.

Select three activities to prioritize for this week.

1.
2.
3.

Be kind to yourself,
dear—to your innocent
follies. Forget any sounds or
touch you knew that did not
help you dance. You will come
to see that all evolves us.

RUMI

HEALTHY-HABIT WORKBOOK

STEP 4
Belonging

AFFIRMATION:

**My breath guides me
back home to Infinite Love.**

HEART-CENTERING

Begin by breathing in and out slowly and deeply three times. You can use a count of five as you breathe in and five as you breathe out; this is a good slow and steady pace. Continue breathing at a comfortable rate. Feel the ground beneath you as our planet holds you safely.

Feel your breath flowing smoothly and evenly over your upper chest area. Allow your breathing to create harmony, flow, and ease in your body, mind, and soul.

SELF-CARING

Go with the flow and ease of nature's balance and rhythm. Fill your heart with gratitude for nature's grace and effortless beauty.

Now continue to breathe in a way that feels comfortable.

> **Belonging is the transformative step that nourishes Loving connection with source, self, and others.**
>
> MICHELLE PECK

HEALTHY-HABIT CHECK-IN

Select three habits to focus on this week.

1. Healthy Eating

This week, I will take several moments to think about where my food comes from. I will consistently give gratitude to my food for providing energy to my body.

2. Social and Friend Interactions

The next time I encounter a negative friend, I will focus on my control of the situation and use more positive self-talk.

3. Learning New Things

Learning contributes to my personal development and growth mindset. I will read one new book this week.

4. Optimism

Since positive thoughts and discussions help the brain release feel-good hormones, I will reframe three negative thoughts with positive ones this week. This way, I am nurturing myself, and I will feel better.

5. Managing Stress

Stress harms my learning capacity, performance, sleep, physical and mental health, and substance usage. I will do a heart-centering practice when I feel stress approaching.

INTENTIONS

INTENTION:

Whenever _____
(situation arises), I will respond by _____
_____

I can ask for anything. What am I asking the Universe for?
_____
_____

OPTIMIZING PLAN:

I will do _____
for this amount of time: _____
in this place: _____
starting _____ **and**
repeating every _____

IF-THEN PLAN:

If _____
then I will remain flexible and instead _____
_____

· PART III ·
Well-Being

Start with the roots to understand how a flower grows
and connects to the garden. Start with the petals,
and you will never know the flower's richness,
nor will you recognize the garden.

MICHELLE PECK

Everything you see
has its roots in the
unseen world. The forms may
change, yet the essence remains
the same. Every wonderful sight
will vanish, every sweet word will
fade, but do not be disheartened. The
source they come from is eternal,
growing, branching out, giving
new life and new joy.

RUMI

THE HISTORY OF *Caring*

Maybe you are searching among the branches for what only appears in the roots. —Rumi

Our ancestors sat around cookfires as they shared stories, which is why stories are so powerful. Storytelling comes from our inheritance. Just imagine the sense of community sitting around the fire, cooking, sharing food, and telling stories.

Around 5,000 years ago, health and caring were first written about in the Vedic texts (Vedanta). In Ayurvedic Medicine (the science of life), there was no separation of mind-body-soul; it was a sophisticated and integrated system (see Figure 2).

SELF-CARING

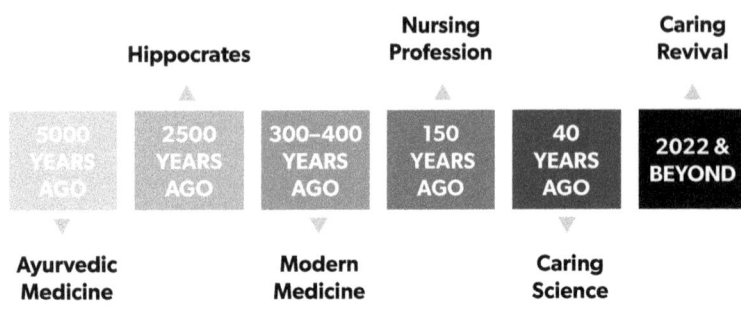

Figure 2. Academy of Well-Being Caring Timeline

Around 2,500 years ago, Hippocrates and many great minds enriched science, and what we know as modern medicine emerged around 300–400 years ago. But unlike the integrated system of the past, the predominant focus was on what we could understand, see, do, and measure (body and body-mind).

> **Put the patient in the best condition for nature to act.**
> FLORENCE NIGHTINGALE

Nursing emerged around 150 years ago, closely following the ways of modern medicine (body and body-mind). But some nurses used integrated systems like Florence Nightingale, whom I call my "nursing mother." Nightingale wrote about the influence of nature as the healer and about health, requiring that we use all our powers to be well.[1]

Caring Science started emerging around forty years ago, and just like the science of life, it is an integrated system. With reflective practice and evolved awareness, Unitary Caring Science provides an advanced guide for humans to live in ways that are more evolved, conscious, and literate.[2]

During the Caring Revival, I hope humanity will learn to fully embrace well-being. Caring for ourselves can be a powerful and enjoyable experience by connecting the science of life to modern science to Caring Science.

Have you ever been afraid of how life is playing out?

A person I'll call Brian was working as a nurse in a hospital critical care unit for two years. I could tell something was off, so I asked the best question I knew: "What is most on your heart today?" As I listened, his story gracefully unfolded like a big blanket tucked away in a storage box up in the attic.

Disconnection, tasks, and duties were stacking up. Brian would repeatedly look at the clock during work hours, counting down the minutes for work to end. The connections he once had with his patients and coworkers were quickly diminishing. Brian was now judging patients and casting blame for what they had done to themselves to wind up in the hospital. Brian was stuck and was burning out quickly.

But Brian had an ardent desire to become like he was when he had first decided to become a nurse—excited, courageous, enthusiastic, and connected. As I listened to Brian using non-judgment, gratitude, and love, his courage and vulnerability opened in the safe space created between us. Brian entered his doorway to belonging, where his creativity and opportunity for change awaited.

I always see the same glistening reflected in the eyes when somebody discovers the wisdom of their inner genius.

Brian also knew he could come to me for peer support because he knew that disconnection had also happened to me at the beginning of my nursing career. He also knew that I learned how to overcome it. So Brian was aspiring to find a new way.

The door of belonging is locked with disconnection and unlocks with connection.

As Brian stepped through the doorway of belonging, he chose a few new ways to connect back to the passion he once had. He started using heart-centering techniques whenever he got stressed, attended peer support groups, and committed to lifelong learning.

Feelings of disconnection cause most of the common symptoms in the real world. The solution is simple—connect back by activating our inner genius. Sitting in a safe space of non-judgment will support and rekindle the power of connection. We can also create this space with others. One way is to ask another caring person to listen to us without trying to fix our problems, and another way is through a peer-support group-healing circle. A group in coherence is a potent way for connecting back in. There is implicit order as consciousness unfolds everything, which arises in participation among us rather than separately.[3]

Brian reconnected the day I listened compassionately. Connection is activated with courage and by stepping through the doorway of belonging. Brian continued to grow his inner resources and in two months was recruiting other nurses to learn about what he had found. Brian went forward on his path by being a role model for those working in his environment. He no longer counted down the minutes for his shift to end. Instead, he spent extra time cultivating new connections and sharing his newfound passions at work.

Brian's rewards were: reconnection, courage, and stepping through the doorway of belonging.

Many people desire better care for themselves and humanity. The excellent news is well-being, self-growth, and caring are no longer a mystery. Our highest potential is accessible and achievable. To live the best version of ourselves, we nurture mind, body, and soul connection.

PERSONAL POWER POINTS

1 · *Self-awareness is an internal relationship to wholeness.*
2 · *Courage and belonging are connective and promote ease and wellness, moving us in the opposite direction of disease and illness.*
3 · *After nurturing our well-being, self-growth, and caring potential, we will help others tremendously.*

Embracing OURSELVES

*Place importance on yourself.
Everything reflects who you are. It's where you focus your
attention that matters. —Michelle Peck*

*I*n 2008, I was sitting at my shared desk in a local nursing facility. It was late, and I had just finished eating my bland take-out dinner while typing twenty client visit notes. My cell phone rang as if on cue—another doctor needing assistance.

Doc said something surprising. "Michelle, I'm concerned about you; you need to start taking better care of yourself." I was immediately enraged. I had just pulled a twelve-hour day, and this was what I got? Not a thank you for diligently caring for everyone.

SELF-CARING

It took me several years before I realized that Doc only cared about my well-being. Initially, I could not hear Doc's advice because he had disturbed me with his opinion. Doc was the first to bring caring for myself to my attention. But back then, I had no idea how to listen to and be lifted by my inner self; so instead, I blamed the messenger. Unfortunately, this drained my energy, blocked my healing ability, and added more symptoms to my list of complaints.

By this time, my coughing from digestion issues was relentless. The peppermint-smelling cream I had discovered for my neck during childhood was slathered all over my upper back and across my throbbing forehead multiple times a day. My shoulders hurt so badly that wearing necklaces or my white coat for more than thirty minutes was unbearable, so instead of carrying my stethoscope around my neck, I stuffed it into a purse strapped around my waist.

Deep down I knew Doc was right, but it still took me years to fully realize this because of the blame I cast his way when he said his words. My reaction stemmed from my lack of understanding about caring for myself, and back then I didn't know about the negative health consequences of casting blame.

Self-Caring is not selfish. It's self-bliss. –Sage Taylor Kingsley

EMBRACING OURSELVES

Self-Caring provides us with the emotional strength to be fully present when other people need to depend on us. When we're able to take care of ourselves as we would our best friend or family member, caring for others becomes more accessible—and everybody will notice that difference too.

Are you struggling to be kind to yourself?

Self-kindness is a powerful tool to help overcome negative thoughts and feelings. It's the path to feel happier and more fulfilled in our lives. When we practice self-kindness, we become our own best friend.

Some examples of self-kindness are:

- Treat yourself with understanding when things don't go as planned or when you make a mistake.
- Learn not to judge yourself for feeling sad, anxious, or angry—because everyone does!

The good news is that practicing self-kindness daily helps build stronger relationships with ourselves and others.

Self-kindness is a path towards achieving success in all areas of life.

SELF-CARING

Here are my five favorite self-kindness tips:

1. You deserve self-kindness.
2. Self-kindness is not selfish.
3. Self-kindness is healthy.
4. Gift yourself the self-kindness you deserve.
5. The only person to approve of you is you.

We all deserve to be our own best friends, and to be mindful of our mental, emotional, spiritual, and physical health by giving ourselves time off from work or other obligations when needed. Practice Self-Caring techniques like heart-centering, mindfulness, journaling, or going out with friends without feeling guilty about it. Give ourselves the self-kindness we deserve after doing something good for someone else just because it feels good! Build confidence and trust in life decisions by accepting who we are—flaws included—instead of trying to force perfection.

One of the most underrated yet powerful tools we have at our disposal is self-kindness.

When practiced regularly, self-kindness can help us feel happier, more content, and more connected, regardless of what life throws our way. I hope these before-to-after examples nurture self-kindness, self-awareness, non-judgment, and self-love in your life.

EMBRACING OURSELVES

Before-to-After Self-Kindness Refocusing Techniques:

- *Before:* You're tired of being hard on yourself. You know you deserve better, but it's hard to be nice to yourself when you don't feel good about yourself.

  After: Imagine treating yourself with the same kindness and thoughtfulness that your best friend would. Wouldn't that make a big difference in how you feel?

- *Before:* You're tired of feeling that you should be better. You feel that you're not good enough and that there is always something more to do, someone else to please, or some other way to improve yourself.

  After: Imagine being kinder to yourself and being gentle with your thoughts and feelings instead of focusing on mistakes or imperfections.

- *Before:* You're tired of beating yourself up when you make a mistake. You've tried to be more forgiving, but it never works for you!

  After: Imagine learning how to forgive your mistakes. It's not easy, but with practice, you can learn to stop the negative self-talk that was keeping you from achieving your goals.

SELF-CARING

Self-kindness is a simple practice that can change our lives in big ways. It's about treating ourselves with care, love, and respect—the same way you would treat others if they needed help and support.

Are you tired of living in a way that isn't true to yourself?

Self-awareness is your inner reflection. We know what's best for us, but it can be hard to find the time and energy to put our needs first. If this sounds familiar, then self-awareness is a solution. We're all busy with work, family, friends, and other commitments, but we can't serve from an empty cup.

Here are some examples of shifting focus to grow self-awareness.

Before-to-After Self-Awareness Refocusing Techniques:

- *Before:* You're tired of feeling that you can't do anything right. You feel that everyone is judging you and that no one likes you.

    After: Imagine seeing yourself through the eyes of someone who loves and accepts you, someone who sees you fully, not as society has told them.

- *Before:* You're tired of the patterns you notice in your life and behavior.

EMBRACING OURSELVES

After: Imagine having a new sense of self-awareness and understanding about how your actions affect others. You make better choices for yourself and those around you.

- *Before:* You're tired of being so self-conscious about your body. You want to be able to wear whatever you want without worrying about what other people think.

After: Imagine feeling confident and comfortable in your skin, no matter what you're wearing or how much you weigh.

Self-worth is not based on society's opinions about our looks or abilities. Instead, it's measured by how much love and acceptance we have for ourselves.

I hope that we all find a way to see ourselves one day through loving eyes and open hearts.

The only person whose opinion matters in this life is yours. In a world full of people who love themselves, we would no longer have to suffer from the debilitating effects of self-hatred. We would be confident and happy with our bodies just as they are because everyone else accepts them too. Imagine a place where you don't feel like an outsider for being different—a place where your weight, skin color, age,

SELF-CARING

physical or mental abilities, or height don't define how beautiful you are. Society just hasn't caught up yet.

Here are some examples of growing self-love and how to shift your looking glass to a more helpful view.

Before-to-After Self-Love Refocusing Techniques:

- *Before:* You're tired of feeling that you don't love yourself enough. You want to feel good about who you are, but it's hard when all your friends and family keep telling you that you aren't good enough.

  After: Imagine a world where everyone loves themselves just the way they are—a world where people treat each other with kindness and respect, no matter size or shape.

- *Before:* You know that self-love is important, but it's so hard to do!

  After: Imagine loving yourself just the way you are, loving your body and all its imperfections, and loving your mind and all its quirks. Loving every part of who you are, even the parts that aren't perfect or easy to love.

Do you ever judge yourself?

EMBRACING OURSELVES

When we judge ourselves, it can lead to low self-esteem and sadness. We often don't realize that the negative thoughts about ourselves are just a result of our judgment. It is essential to recognize these judgments and shift them to avoid becoming destructive.

Before-to-After Self-Judgment Refocusing Techniques:

- *Before:* I am never good enough.

  After: I am more than enough; everybody has some setbacks. But I am growing from my experiences.

- *Before:* Why even try, I will never get those results because I'm not smart enough.

  After: Imagine having a friend who is always there for you no matter what, always willing to listen without judgment or criticism, and encourages you to do your best. Now imagine being that friend for yourself.

- *Before:* You keep telling yourself the same story over and over again. You've tried to stop judging yourself, but you just can't seem to do it!

  After: Imagine a world where you are free from the self-judgment that holds you back and can create anything you desire.

SELF-CARING

We may be great at so many things, but can't stop being our own worst critic. It's time to change that and let ourselves off the hook. We all have moments when we're not feeling our best or are just having a difficult day. We can live in a direction that supports well-being, self-growth, and caring by refocusing on a more positive perspective.

Now let's explore forgiveness, another powerful way to activate a higher potential.

It's hard to forgive ourselves, especially when we think we've screwed up royally. But guess what? It's time to start forgiving ourselves because self-forgiveness is good for our health, improves relationships, and makes us happier overall. Admittedly, it's not easy to find self-forgiveness, but it's necessary to live a happy life without carrying blame towards ourselves.

There is no reason not to give ourselves forgiveness.

The act of forgiving ourselves can be just as important as forgiving others. Forgiving helps relieve stress and anxiety so we can find peace within. We all make mistakes. We all have regrets. The ability to forgive ourselves for wrongdoings is not always easy, but is always worth it.

EMBRACING OURSELVES

Here are my five favorite steps toward self-forgiveness:

1. Acknowledge your mistake. Own up to it.
2. Don't dwell on what happened. Focus on moving forward on your journey.
3. Be gentle. Forgiveness does not happen overnight.
4. Forgive yourself, then forgive yourself repeatedly.
5. Learn from your experience and move on by embracing your wholeness.

We're only human. We will make mistakes and have regrets from time to time. The key is being able to forgive ourselves for wrongdoings. So if you find yourself feeling down on yourself today or any other given day, I hope you remember these ways to help you feel better.

PERSONAL POWER POINTS

1. *One of the most underrated yet powerful tools we have at our disposal is self-kindness.*
2. *Self-worth is not based on society's opinions about our looks or abilities, it's measured by how much love and acceptance we have for ourselves.*
3. *Forgiving ourselves relieves stress and nurtures the potential for living in grace, ease, and flow.*

MINDFUL GRATITUDE JOURNAL

STEP 5

Embrace

AFFIRMATION:

All I need is here, now, in the gift of the present moment.

Pause after each question. Answer by asking, "What is most on my heart today?"

How are my surroundings supporting me?

SELF-CARING

What are the barriers between me and reaching my highest and best potential?

From what have I disconnected?

What did I try to fill this disconnect with?

What lessons am I learning?

How has my journey changed my ability to connect with other people?

How can I nurture self-kindness in everyday life?

Gratitude

Three aspects of my personality or body that I am grateful for are:

1.

2.

3.

List three things this week that were beautiful. Make sure to include some description about how the things looked, felt, smelled, tasted, and sounded.

1.

2.

3.

**Grace comes to forgive
and then forgive again.**

RUMI

HEALTHY-HABIT WORKBOOK

STEP 5
Embrace

AFFIRMATION:

**My potential is infinite,
and everything helps me grow.**

HEART-CENTERING

Begin by breathing in and out slowly and deeply three times. You can use a count of five as you breathe in and five as you breathe out; this is a good slow and steady pace. Then feel the ground beneath you as our planet holds you safely.

Imagine your breath flowing in and out of your upper chest as you continue to breathe. Allow your breath to flow in and out smoothly, slowly, and deeply.

SELF-CARING

Take a scan of your body. Make a note of areas that feel tight or tense. Feel your in-breath flowing into each tight area stored in your body and your out-breath releasing the tension. Breathe gratitude into the tight spots and allow them to release with the out-breath.

Now continue to breathe in a way that feels comfortable.

> **Embrace yourself with self-kindness and amplify well-being.**
>
> MICHELLE PECK

HEALTHY-HABIT CHECK-IN

Select three habits to focus on this week.

1. Healthy Eating

This week, I will slow down during my favorite meal of the day to enjoy each bite. I will appreciate the smell, color, temperature, texture, and flavor of the food.

2. Exercising

My body needs to move. When I feel the stress wave approaching this week, I will get active and move into calm and comfort instead of letting it crash down on me.

3. Rest and Sleep

There are times when it may be difficult for me to get adequate sleep. I will commit to meditating to recover my brain whenever my sleep is disrupted.

4. Variety and Challenge

Boredom is a destructive process that negatively impacts my health. This week, when I feel bored, I will shift into a curious mindset and discover something new.

5. Social and Friend Interactions

This week, I will prioritize my friends and make sure to reserve time to have some fun.

INTENTIONS

INTENTION:

Whenever _____
(situation arises), I will respond by _____
_____

I can ask for anything. What am I asking the Universe for?
_____
_____

OPTIMIZING PLAN:

I will do _____
for this amount of time: _____
in this place: _____
starting _____ **and**
repeating every _____

IF-THEN PLAN:

If _____
then I will remain flexible and instead _____
_____

Inspire & Jump
AGAIN

Belonging lives inside me. Whenever I feel rejected, I look inside of myself. After I accept myself fully, healing flows naturally. With each obstacle in my path, I will jump and jump again until I fly at last. —Michelle Peck

My journey continues forward, even though I still meet some obstacles in my way. Each time I jump a mountain I grow stronger until one day I will fly with blazing wings like a Phoenix rising above the ashes.

If we are standing on the beach without a surfboard and cannot swim when the waves crash down on us, that's just like holding onto stress. However, if we focus on the wave differently, we can switch to a win by empowering personal resilience (to jump again). The process of resiliency involves growth enhancement strategies, stress management, and the ability to use skills and inner resources to respond to ongoing stressors effectively.[1] In other words, we can learn to change our perspectives to being champion surfers and not victims of a limited view, to surf the giant stress wave in alignment and flow with nature.

> **You have escaped the cage. Your wings are stretched out. Now fly.**
>
> RUMI

When we fall face-first in the mud, we can get up and jump out if we have high personal resiliency. But even more impressive, if we grow our resiliency, we can use obstacles and adversities as springboards to reach a higher level than where we were before the disruption. Seven core learnable characteristics reside in highly resilient people: (1) calm, non-dogmatic, innovative thinking, (2) decisive action, (3) tenacity, (4) interpersonal connectedness, (5) self-control, (6) honesty, and (7) a positive, optimistic life perspective.[2]

A mountain of opportunity will appear many times during our lifetime. We can walk or crawl away. We can ignore it and pretend we don't see it. We can feel defeated and sit or lay facedown in the mud. But we can also learn to jump the mountain. By learning to jump, each time a new mountain appears, we have a greater power to jump over it too.

Our desire and attitude impact personal resiliency.

Rumi shares the poem "Guest House" to remind us to meet our thoughts and emotions passing through with courage, warmth, and respect.

> *This being human is a guest house.*
> *Every morning a new arrival.*
>
> *A joy, a depression, a meanness,*
> *some momentary awareness comes*
> *as an unexpected visitor.*
>
> *Welcome and entertain them all!*
> *Even if they're a crowd of sorrows,*
> *who violently sweep your house*
> *empty of its furniture,*
> *still, treat each guest honorably.*
> *He may be clearing you out*
> *for some new delight.*
>
> *The dark thought, the shame, the malice,*
> *meet them at the door laughing,*
> *and invite them in.*
>
> *Be grateful for whoever comes,*
> *because each has been sent*
> *as a guide from beyond.*

I prefer to focus on challenge as an opportunity to increase personal resiliency, which leads to more growth, balance, and flourishing. Focus on viewing challenges, obstacles, and adversity as opportunities for growing your abilities to jump higher.

There are four dimensions of personal resilience—physical, emotional, mental, and spiritual.[3] However, *most people only focus on the physical*—building flexibility, endurance, and strength.

We must develop all four dimensions of personal resilience.

EMOTIONAL FLEXIBILITY

How often do we find ourselves stuck in our emotions? Whether it's anger, sadness, or fear, we can get hooked on our negative feelings, and they dictate how we behave and how we see the world. Emotional flexibility means using a range of emotions, adopting positive feelings, and learning self-regulation to nurture relationships. Our emotional flexibility allows us to move through our feelings more quickly, with less reactivity and more responsiveness. When we are emotionally flexible, we can stay centered despite challenging situations. We are also better equipped to connect with others from a place of gratitude rather than judgment.

We all want to feel better. But if we're struggling with our emotions, it's time to take a deep breath and start the process of changing how we see ourselves and others. Emotional flexibility means easily adapting by shifting into a more responsive emotional state. When emotionally flexible, we are better equipped for life's challenges and can nurture more fulfilling and sustainable relationships.

MENTAL FLEXIBILITY

Mental flexibility is one of the most underrated life skills. It's what allows us to adapt to change, see different perspectives, and deepen creativity. And it's a skill that we all need now more than ever. Our world is constantly evolving, and we must change with it.

Ways to grow mental flexibility include:

- Mindfulness and gratitude practices.
- Growing your attention span.
- Keeping an optimistic view.
- Considering many points of view.

All these aspects are mental flexibility skills that we can grow to help us thrive in the world.

SPIRITUAL FLEXIBILITY

As we learn to commit to personal core values, we also will grow in tolerance for the beliefs of others and further develop our intuitive abilities. To maintain balance and increase personal resilience, we can't be rigid and fixed, polarized, or view this as right and that as wrong. Flexibility resides in between.

We all can adapt, withstand, and rebound from a disruption to our natural balance (or homeostasis). It is desirable to live in flow for health, wellness, and healing and grow the ability to adjust back to flow easily. Polarizing (creating absolutes) is where everything crashes down on us. Flow means guiding ourselves to the center of the opposites, neutrality. Polarized opposites will keep us stuck.

The field of neutrality is flow. Nature is neutral.

We all need to be more flexible in our lives. And if you've ever been caught up in a Chinese finger trap, then you know just how difficult it can be to find that flexibility when your fingers are stuck by pulling them apart, and the only thing keeping them from being free is joining them together.

We control the flexibility of our responses when we come together in neutrality instead of separating with opposition.

Do you find yourself constantly striving for excellence, fearing failure, or never fully satisfied with your accomplishments?

A research review found that the most substantial psychological factors in easing the experience of failure and emotional dysfunction were:

1. Lower levels of perfectionism.
2. Higher self-esteem.
3. Positive attributional style (explained more below).[4]

We all have moments of failure. But the most important thing is how we react to them. Lowering our perfectionism, increasing self-esteem, and adopting a more positive attributional style can help us tremendously. Now let's explore these three psychological factors some more.

A lot of people struggle with perfectionism. For many people, the pressure to be perfect is intense. For some, this pressure can lead to anxiety and depression. In addition, it can result in obsessive perfectionism that can have destructive consequences. While striving for excellence is an admirable goal, perfectionism can go too far and become a dangerous obsession.

If you find yourself constantly striving for excellence without ever feeling fully satisfied with your accomplishments, know that there are people who understand what you're going through. I was once a perfectionism-driven young woman who struggled because of my constant need to do more than the next person to feel good about myself. Nowadays, I am happy enough just being, flaws included, and I want everyone else to have the same opportunity for happiness too. Striving to be good enough is much healthier than striving to be perfect.

Higher self-esteem is a key to happiness.

Do you know that feeling when you don't feel your best? You're not sure what it is, but something just doesn't feel right. As a result, confidence is down, and it's hard to push through the day. We might even compare ourselves to others and feel that we're coming up short. Chances are if this sounds familiar, then self-esteem could use a boost. Fortunately, there are plenty of ways to build our confidence and raise self-esteem.

When we have high self-esteem, we feel good about ourselves and lives. We feel confident and know that we can achieve anything we set our minds to. Low self-esteem, on the other hand, can be incredibly damaging. It can lead to depression, anxiety, and a host of other problems. So how do we raise self-esteem?

Here are my three favorite tips for boosting self-esteem:

1. Be gentle with yourself. Don't be too hard on yourself when you make a mistake. Everyone makes mistakes sometimes. It's human nature!
2. Forgive yourself and move on because this is essential for your self-esteem.
3. Allow yourself to shine because you deserve it!

Do you tend to focus on your strengths and positive qualities?

If so, you have what psychologists call a "positive attributional style." This means that we tend to give ourselves and others the benefit of the doubt and see the good in any situation. A positive attributional style can lead to greater happiness and success in life.

Three examples of a *positive* attributional style are:

1. I failed because this project was challenging.
2. I know that next time I will do better.
3. I failed at this project, but I am good at many other things.

Three examples of a *negative* attributional style are:

1. I failed because I am no good.
2. I always fail, so why should I even try?
3. I fail at everything; failing this time was no surprise.

SELF-CARING

We can focus on multiple factors to feel good about our lives even when things don't go as planned. However, most successful people have one thing in common—they don't give up when faced with failure. If we strive for perfectionism at every turn, it will be much harder to see progress and feel good about ourselves.

PERSONAL POWER POINTS

1. *When faced with stress, obstacles, or challenges, our reaction determines our ability to bounce back.*
2. *Don't give up; failure often means a better opportunity is waiting for us.*
3. *Strive for good enough, not perfect.*

Gratitude, Balance
& ENERGY IN MOTION

*Wherever water flows, life flourishes.
Wherever tears fall, divine mercy is shown.* —Rumi

The dark side of me is constantly pushing. I'm tired, yet I want to be good. It's easy sometimes, but when I get pushed too far, that voice comes out. Somebody makes a comment, or something happens, and bad things spill out of my mouth. We all have that little monster inside us.

We are not just a mind; we are also the intelligence of our whole being. Our intelligence flows from every pore throughout our bodies. The entire body fills with the power of our intelligence. We can sense it when we meditate or relax and let go. Reality is created by how we think, feel, and act.

SELF-CARING

Emotions should flow like waves in the ocean. What we cast out is what we catch. For example, we can cast out blessings to catch blessings or curses to catch curses.

> **If your thought is a rose, you are a rose garden; and if it is a thistle, you are fuel for the fire.**
>
> RUMI

Imagine a giant fishing pole with a dangling line and a sharp hook. Now think of emotions as energy in motion. When we feel an emotion, we place it on the sharp hook and watch as it swings side to side. Then we cast our line out into the universal ocean. Heavy emotions weigh down the line. Other emotions feel as light as air and are easy to cast and pull back in. Whatever we cast out is what we reel in.

> **The world is a mountain, in which your words are echoed back to you.**
>
> RUMI

To discover how it feels to know if your emotion is heavy or light, ask your body. All feelings will fit into two big jars of either light (comfort) or heavy (discomfort). The feeling of being "weighed down" or "carrying the weight of the world on your shoulders" is real—stress stores in the body as heavy density. Once we surf the gigantic stress wave, we will notice how light and comfortable our body feels. When we cast out good vibes to the universal sea, good vibes are what we will catch.

GRATITUDE, BALANCE & ENERGY IN MOTION

We are energetic beings. Our vibrations are measurable and can be felt by those around us. Even a dog knows if we are having a good or dreadful day without us having to explain it to them because they sense our vibration. Living with a balanced body-mind-soul means gently rebalancing back when our vibration goes out of balance.

> **Gratitude is the wine for the soul. Go on. Get drunk.**
> RUMI

As we polish our mirrors, we will notice that emotions flow just like the waves of the ocean. They rise and fall and come and go. They are dynamic and change, sometimes even second to second in pressure-filled situations. If we hold onto heavy emotions, they will drain our energy, weigh us down, build up, and create density (dis-ease), the opposite of ease.

Getting stuck with heavy emotions does not serve us or anyone for that matter. Instead of exhausting ourselves, we can try being aware of our energy levels. We can drain ourselves in many ways. Try avoiding what drains energy and favoring what naturally boosts energy.

A research review described numerous psychological and physical well-being benefits from experiencing positive emotions.[1] To live a flourishing life think flourishing in spirit, flourishing in mind, and flourishing in connection.

Focusing on gratitude brings us into flow and empowers our potential.

Think of a river. The rocky banks can snag and stop a canoe. Being in balance means flowing with the river. While we cannot control the river's flow, we can focus on counterbalancing what is holding us back and get back into the flow. We can focus on what is right in our lives and what makes us grateful just as quickly as we can on what is wrong or who wronged us. Placing our focus on wrongdoings and wrongdoers will drain our potential (keep our canoe stuck).

> **Wear gratitude like a cloak, and it will feed every corner of your life.**
>
> RUMI

Where we choose to focus is what we will grow.

When terrible things happen to us, they can throw off our balance for a while. It is impossible to control the river. It is impossible to control the waves of the ocean. Flow with the water—and wellness, growth, caring, health, and healing come naturally. This is the path toward lasting joy in work and living.

The ocean is a great analogy for life because waves constantly come in and out. When we are at the top of one wave, it's time to prepare for our next experience. We have an incredible power within ourselves. When we focus on our highest and best wellness, self-growth, and caring abilities, we gain a tremendous advantage.

PERSONAL POWER POINTS

1 · *How we react always matters.*
2 · *Gratitude brings balance, empowerment, and flow.*
3 · *Replacing heavy polarizing emotions with neutral and grateful ones keeps energy flowing like a river.*

Out beyond ideas
of wrongdoing and
rightdoing, there is a field.
I'll meet you there.
When the soul lies down
in that grass, the world is
too full to talk about.

RUMI

MINDFUL GRATITUDE JOURNAL

STEP 6

Balance

AFFIRMATION:

I create balance by taking a few breaths and focusing on whatever I am grateful for.

Pause after each question. Answer by asking, "What is most on my heart today?"

How emotionally flexible am I? The areas in my life where I tend to hold on too tightly are:

1.

SELF-CARING

2.

3.

4.

5.

What curses am I shifting to blessings?

1.

2.

3.

4.

Example: I used to hold resentment for always having to listen to my friend's problems. Instead, I will focus on my blessing of being a good listener during these troubling times.

MINDFUL GRATITUDE JOURNAL · STEP 6: BALANCE

How did I learn to deal (or not deal) with stress at an early age?

What coping strategies did I learn from my family or culture?

SELF-CARING

What was the last stressful situation I encountered? Did I disconnect from the problem, buckle down, or power through? Or did the stress crash down on me?

What will I try the next time a stressful situation surfaces?

Draft a paragraph about a time that I failed.

Did my paragraph use a positive or negative attributional style? Why?

Rewrite my paragraph of failure while focusing on a positive attributional style.

SELF-CARING

Create a list of skills that I want to learn or continue to improve.

1.
2.
3.
4.
5.
6.
7.
8.
9.
10.

Describe three ways I envision improving the skills I desire to grow.

1.

2.

3.

MINDFUL GRATITUDE JOURNAL · STEP 6: BALANCE

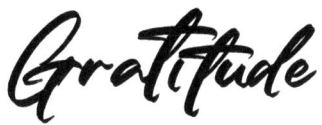

Describe a time when I was extremely grateful.

Set a timer for 90 seconds and list my favorite simple pleasures in life, everyday things that make me happy.

1.
2.
3.
4.
5.
6.
7.
8.
9.
10.
11.
12.
13.

HEALTHY-HABIT WORKBOOK

STEP 6
Balance

AFFIRMATION:

I maintain balance and persevere using great tenacity and determination.

HEART-CENTERING

Begin by breathing in and out slowly and deeply three times. You can use a count of five as you breathe in and five as you breathe out; this is a good slow and steady pace. Then, place your feet on the ground and pull safety and strength up from our planet.

Imagine your breath flowing in and out of your upper chest as you continue to breathe at a comfortable pace. Envision a time in your life when you were extremely grateful. Notice how you feel as you sit in this time of gratitude.

SELF-CARING

Now breathe this feeling of gratitude deeply into your upper chest area and relax into your body, allowing gratitude to fill you up.

Feel the gratitude as you continue to breathe into your upper chest area.

Gratitude and safety from our Universe surround you as you flow with nature in harmony and balance.

Now continue to breathe in a way that feels comfortable.

Balance creates harmony with all that surrounds me.

MICHELLE PECK

HEALTHY-HABIT CHECK-IN

Select three habits to focus on this week.

1. Healthy Eating

This week, I will pay attention to eating more fruits and vegetables because their polyphenols and antioxidants boost my brain's ability.

2. Exercising

This week, I will focus on finding one new recreational way to keep my body moving.

3. Rest and Sleep

I will look up various sleep hygiene practices to create my ideal bedtime routine.

4. Optimism

To build my resilience, I will keep up a consistent effort to be optimistic. I am an optimist!

5. Learning New Things

I will set aside five minutes a day to learn something new and exciting.

SELF-CARING

INTENTIONS

INTENTION:

Whenever _____
(situation arises), I will respond by _____
_____

I can ask for anything. What am I asking the Universe for?
_____
_____

OPTIMIZING PLAN:

I will do _____
for this amount of time: _____
in this place: _____
starting _____ **and**
repeating every _____

IF-THEN PLAN:

If _____
then I will remain flexible and instead _____
_____

WELL-BEING,
We Are Blooming

*Your right and left hand are opposites.
But when you bring your hands together, they align in unity—
harmony with all creation. —Michelle Peck*

A person I'll call Kim began aggressively criticizing my parenting. My feelings grew stronger with every word that came out of her mouth. Finally, my heart started pounding, trying to escape out of my chest. This intense feeling was a reminder not to get lost in the moment and to stay aware enough to ground me while being open-minded enough to hear Kim's perspective.

I used the power of my breath and reminded myself to take a pause. As I focused on my breathing, I made it slower and deeper than before, making space for gratitude to fill me up like water filling an empty cup, and then I decided not to say anything for a while. Instead, I listened attentively without judgment. Finally, I came into the field of neutrality by saying to myself, "Kim is on her perfect path, just like me. And at this moment, this is how Kim feels."

Listening without interruption made it so easy; suddenly, my newfound power felt terrific—like taking off running after someone who has always seemed far ahead but is now within reach. Then finally, my mirror was crystal clear, no more rust, and I was capable of reflecting Kim's wholeness to her. I no longer reflected as a dusty, rusty mirror. Instead, I had learned to come fully into compassion.

We can't always be grateful for what happens, but we can always choose our response.

I knew that the longer I reflected Kim's wholeness to her, the more likely she could recognize something more than her perception of my parenting. Shortly after her intense episode of emotion, she apologized and gave me a supportive hug!

When I first began to train as a coach, one of the most challenging skills for me was identifying and releasing feelings of judgment. However, after practicing over time, nonjudgment and neutrality became natural.

Each time a sense of criticism or judgment comes on, I direct my thinking back to my inner resources, and I choose to grow connections. For example, one great guide helped me learn how deep listening and a compassionate heart will calm someone's fears. The artistry happens by not critiquing another's perspective but instead focusing on how everyone is doing their best in any given moment. Raising your frequency by breathing gratitude into your heart can also increase the frequency of others. But on the other hand, if you meet someone while carrying a low-frequency feeling like fear, blame, anger, guilt, or resentment, your low vibration when paired with theirs can worsen or escalate the situation.

Fear is disconnection. Compassion is connection.

Fear tricks you into thinking that you are protecting yourself. Flourishing can only happen through courage, belonging, and letting go of fear. Once you walk through the doorway of belonging, feeling lighter, freer, and living at a higher frequency, you too will hold the door open for others.

We all have the needs for belonging and safety. The space created by holding an intention for wellness, growth, caring, and connection allows us to learn more, care about others, heal from past hurts, and grow our relationships. Whenever there's an opportunity to create a space where people feel that they belong, it brings out the best within us too.

The beauty you see in me is a reflection of you. —*Rumi*

It can be hard to find the time and space for ourselves in the real world when we're constantly connected through our phones or computers but feel disconnected from those around us. Sometimes there are just too many miles between two people who care deeply about one another, which makes communicating without any misunderstanding difficult.

Have you ever noticed an automatic sense of safety when we make other people feel that they belong?

We underestimate how much listening in nonjudgment and our presence can help someone, especially if they're struggling in some way. It's hard not to be at peace when we feel surrounded by someone who loves and supports our every move. There is an art to creating a safe space for belonging in any personal or social setting, and our responses can benefit everyone involved.

Every day we are faced with decisions that create better health and wellness. Moment by moment, the choices we make determine our self-growth, wellness, and caring. We all deserve a Self-Caring lifestyle of being blooming!

WELL-BEING, WE ARE BLOOMING

We all have a story worth telling, and others need (and want) to hear ours more than ever right now. So go ahead, create a safe space, and tell them all about yourself with every fiber of your being because there is nothing better than living guided by your inner genius.

You deserve a big hug. And that's what you should do right now: give yourself a hug! And a bonus one from me. It takes courage to focus on well-being, self-growth, and living your Self-Caring Revival.

It's our time to be attractively healthy and full of energy. Congratulations on becoming blooming!

Let's continue to inspire one another and create a better world.

PERSONAL POWER POINTS

1 · *Nurture the harmony and healing power of neutrality.*
2 · *We can choose to grow connections.*
3 · *Everyone benefits when we care for ourselves.*

There is awe and
wonderment at
this moment, and in
wholeness-union-blooming,
you.

MICHELLE PECK

MINDFUL GRATITUDE JOURNAL

STEP 7
Blooming

AFFIRMATION:

I am infinite potential, love in action,
and I celebrate togetherness.

*Pause after each question. Answer by asking,
"What is most on my heart today?"*

How has living Self-Caring changed my relationship with myself?

SELF-CARING

I can care better for others now that I committed to well-being, self-growth, and caring for myself. Describe an opportunity for mentoring someone.

My Blooming

DEEP ROOTS

What nourishes me?

1.

2.

3.

MINDFUL GRATITUDE JOURNAL · STEP 7: BLOOMING

4 ·

5 ·

What hurts my nourishment?

1 ·

2 ·

3 ·

4 ·

5 ·

STEM

What do I stand *for*?

1 ·

2 ·

SELF-CARING

3.

4.

5.

What do I stand *against*?

1.

2.

3.

4.

5.

PETALS

What do I desire to grow more of in my life?

1.

2.

3.

What do I need to step away from to continue blooming?

1.

2.

3.

SELF-CARING

MY SELF-CARING REVIVAL

Looks like:

Tastes like:

Smells like:

Feels like:

Sounds like:

MY GARDEN OF TOGETHERNESS

Looks like:

Tastes like:

Smells like:

Feels like:

Sounds like:

Gratitude

Remember a joyful experience. What were you doing?

How did the situation come to be?

How did your body, mind, and heart feel?

What does it mean to be joyful?

> Every parcel of my being
> is in full bloom.
>
> — RUMI

HEALTHY-HABIT WORKBOOK

STEP 7
Blooming

AFFIRMATION:

My strong and deep roots will
always nourish me.

HEART-CENTERING

Begin by breathing in and out slowly and deeply three times.

Imagine a flower bud tightly closed with a beautiful flower inside. The flower wants to peek out of the impenetrable fortress, but nature has not allowed for this quite yet.

Nurture the flower with your breath. Know that the bloom will open and unfold its petaled tapestry to decorate the world at precisely the right moment. As you breathe gratitude deeply into

SELF-CARING

your upper chest, your flower blooms gently on the out-breath and in flow with nature in this present, perfect moment.

You are this flower. As you open your courage, you walk through the doorway of belonging. You are now blooming and flourishing in the garden of togetherness.

Now continue to breathe in a way that feels comfortable.

> **Well-being enlivens compassion, the highest frequency of love.**
>
> MICHELLE PECK

HEALTHY-HABIT CHECK-IN

Select three habits to focus on this week.

1. Healthy Eating

This week, I will pay attention to eating protein because it helps regulate my mood, thinking ability, memory, and concentration. I will also eat regular and healthy meals because this is important for my gut biome.

2. Exercising

Exercise is good for my body, and it also positively affects my mind. I will focus on enjoying my exercise this week.

3. Making Autonomous Decisions

This week, I will think about somebody I feel grateful for and do something special for them to let them know.

4. Variety and Challenge

I will treat this weekend as if I am on vacation.

5. Social and Friend Interactions

This week, I will make a date with a friend to try something new together and celebrate my well-being!

SELF-CARING

INTENTIONS

INTENTION:

Whenever _____
(situation arises), I will respond by _____
_____

I can ask for anything. What am I asking the Universe for?
_____
_____

OPTIMIZING PLAN:

I will do _____
for this amount of time: _____
in this place: _____
starting _____ **and**
repeating every _____

IF-THEN PLAN:

If _____
then I will remain flexible and instead _____

You are the mirror of divine beauty.

You have no idea how hard I've looked for a gift to bring You. Nothing seemed right. What's the point of bringing gold to the gold mine, or water to the ocean. Everything I came up with was like taking spices to the Orient. It's no good giving my heart and my soul because you already have these. So I've brought you a mirror. Look at yourself and remember me.

RUMI

I am always curious to know more about your experience with this book. Wherever you purchased this book, please consider writing a review.

In gratitude,

Michelle

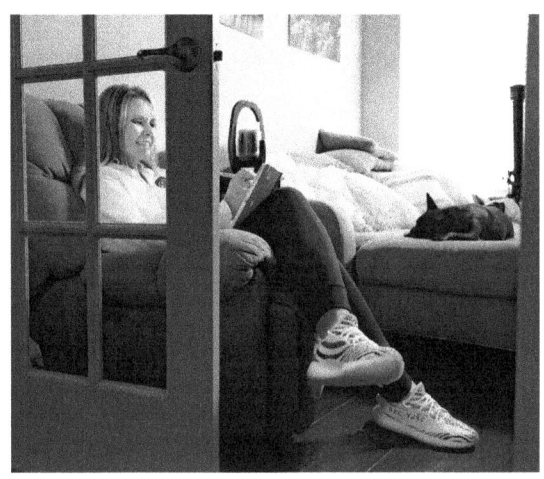

About the Author

MICHELLE PECK has devoted her career to caring for and teaching others as a nurse, public health advocate, and instructor. She grew her caring abilities as a parent and as a nurse practitioner caring for adults at home and at clinics, hospitals, rehabilitation, hospice, memory care, assisted living, and long-term care facilities. An expert nurse, storyteller, coach, and inspirational speaker, she has cared for and taught thousands of people.

As a caring expert and well-being thought leader, she teaches how to first grow in Self-Caring and then how to care for others compassionately.

Peck is a breath of fresh air when it comes to helping people achieve their highest and best potential. She is a Chopra Certified Total Well-being Coach,™ Chopra Health™ Instructor and Chopra Meditation™ Instructor who teaches a holistic way to achieve well-being using Self-Caring, meditation, nutrition, movement, sleep, and healthy emotions. She is also a HeartMath® Certified Trainer and a Watson Caring Science Institute Certified Caritas Coach®. Peck holds a Master of Science in Nursing and Master of Public Health from The University of Texas Health Science Center at Houston. She lives in Texas with her husband, Raul, children, Leon and Nico, and her companion dogs, Vande and Avery.

CONNECT WITH MICHELLE

Please visit the Academy of Well-Being at
www.academyofwellbeing.com
to learn more about our customized corporate and individual well-being courses, programs, and resources.

Endnotes

GETTING STARTED

1. Bernie S. Siegal, *Love, Medicine & Miracles: Lessons Learned About Self-Healing from a Surgeon's Experience with Exceptional Patients* (New York: Harper & Row, 1986).

2. David O. Fakunle, MPH, David T. Thomas, Kathy A. M. Gonzales, Denise C. Vidot, and LaShaune P. Johnson, "What Anansi Did for Us: Storytelling's Value in Equitably Exploring Public Health," *Health Education & Behavior* 48, no. 3 (2021): 352–60. https://doi.org/10.1177/10901981211009741.

3. Joyce B. Perkins, "Watson's Ten Caritas Processes with the Lens of Unitary Human Caring Science," *Nursing Science Quarterly* 34, no. 2 (2021): 157–67. https://doi.org/10.1177/0894318420987176.

4. Rollin McCraty, "New Frontiers in Heart Rate Variability and Social Coherence Research: Techniques, Technologies, and Implications for Improving Group Dynamics and Outcomes," *Frontiers in Public Health* 5 (2017): 267–67. https://doi.org/10.3389/fpubh.2017.00267.

5. Jorina Elbers and Rollin McCraty, "HeartMath Approach to Self-Regulation and Psychosocial Well-Being," *Journal of Psychology in Africa* 30, no. 1 (2020): 69–79. https://doi.org/10.1080/14330237.2020.1712797.

6. Chiara Ruini and Cristina C. Mortara, "Writing Technique across Psychotherapies—from Traditional Expressive Writing to New Positive Psychology Interventions: A Narrative Review," *Journal of Contemporary Psychotherapy* (2021): 1–12. https://doi.org/10.1007/s10879-021-09520-9.

7. Yu Komase, Kazuhiro Watanabe, Daisuke Hori, Kyosuke Nozawa, Yui Hidaka, Mako Iida, Kotaro Imamura, and Norito Kawakami, "Effects of Gratitude Intervention on Mental Health and Well-Being among Workers: A Systematic Review," *Journal of Occupational Health* 63, no. 1 (2021): e12290-e90. https://doi.org/10.1002/1348-9585.12290.

8. Rolf Ekman, Anna Fletcher, Joanna Giota, Axel Eriksson, Bertil Thomas, and Fredrik Bååthe, "A Flourishing Brain in the

ENDNOTES

21st Century: A Scoping Review of the Impact of Developing Good Habits for Mind, Brain, Well-Being, and Learning," *Mind, Brain and Education* in Press (2021). https://doi.org/10.1111/mbe.12305.

9. James Clear, *Atomic Habits: An Easy & Proven Way to Build Good Habits & Break Bad Ones* (New York: Penguin Random House, 2018).

10. Heidi Grant Halvorson, "The If-Then Solution: No Willpower? No Problem (the Science of Success)," *Psychology Today* 44, no. 1 (2011): 48.

ASPIRE & UPGRADE OUR SYSTEMS

1. Cameron G. Ford, Laura G. Kiken, Ilana Haliwa, and Natalie J. Shook, "Negatively Biased Cognition as a Mechanism of Mindfulness: A Review of the Literature," *Current Psychology* (2021). https://doi.org/10.1007/s12144-021-02147-y.

MEET OUR GUIDE

1. Sir Percy Sykes, *Literature and Architecture Under the Mongols* (New York: Routledge, 1915). doi:10.4324/9781315017136-19.

2. Joy Xu, Jo Helen, Leena Noorbhai, Ami Patel, and Amy Li, "Virtual Mindfulness Interventions to Promote Well-Being in Adults: A Mixed-Methods Systematic Review," *Journal of Affective Disorders* (2022/01/04/2022). https://www.sciencedirect.com/science/article/pii/S016503272200026X.

BELONGING BEFORE BEING, KNOWING & DOING

1. Maria Arman, Albertine Ranheim, Kenneth Rydenlund, Patrik Rytterström, and Arne Rehnsfeldt, "The Nordic Tradition of Caring Science: The Works of Three Theorists," *Nursing Science Quarterly* 28, no. 4 (2015): 288–96. https://doi.org/10.1177/0894318415599220.

2. Jean Watson, *Nursing: The Philosophy and Science of Caring* (Boulder, CO: University Press of Colorado, 1985).

3. David R. Hawkins, *The Map of Consciousness Explained: A Proven Energy Scale to Actualize Your Ultimate Potential* (Carlsbad, CA: Hay House, 2020).

4. Jean Watson, *Caring Science as Sacred Science: New Revised Edition* (La Vergne: Lotus Library Watson Caring Science Institute, 2021).

5. Mick Collins, "The Akashic Field and Archetypal Occupations: Transforming Human Potential through

Doing and Being," *World Futures* 67, no. 7 (2011): 453–79. https://doi.org/10.1080/02604027.2011.563190.

6. Ervin Laszlo, Deepak Chopra, and Stanislav Grof, *What Is Reality? The New Map of Cosmos, Consciousness, and Existence* (New York: SelectBooks, Inc., 2016).

THE HISTORY OF CARING

1. Florence Nightingale, *Notes on Nursing: What It Is, and What It Is Not*, Commemorative Edition (Philadelphia: Lippincott, 1992).

2. Sara Horton-Deutsch and Jean Watson, "Ways of Being Knowing Becoming," Chapter 13 In *A Handbook for Caring Science Expanding the Paradigm*, edited by Marilyn Ray, Marlaine Smith, Marian Turkel, Diane Gullett, and Grissel Hernandez-Kertland (New York: Springer Publishing Company, 2019), pp. 189–96.

3. David Bohm, *On Dialogue* (New York: Routledge Great Minds, 2014).

SELF-CARING

INSPIRE & JUMP AGAIN

1. Elyse R. Park, Christina M. Luberto, Emma Chad-Friedman, Lara Traeger, Daniel L. Hall, Giselle K. Perez, Brett Goshe, et al., "A Comprehensive Resiliency Framework: Theoretical Model, Treatment, and Evaluation," *Global Advances in Health and Medicine* 10 (2021): 1–10. https://doi.org/10.1177/21649561211000306.

2. George Everly, Dennis McCormack, and Douglas Strouse, "Seven Characteristics of Highly Resilient People: Insights from Navy SEALs to the 'Greatest Generation,'" *International Journal of Emergency Mental Health* 14, no. 2, (2012): 137–143. https://ssrn.com/abstract=2118935

3. Rollin McCraty and Doc Childre, "Coherence: Bridging Personal, Social, and Global Health," *Alternative Therapies in Health and Medicine* 16, no. 4 (2010): 10–24.

4. Judith Johnson, Maria Panagioti, Jennifer Bass, Lauren Ramsey, and Reema Harrison, "Resilience to Emotional Distress in Response to Failure, Error or Mistakes: A Systematic Review," *Clinical Psychology Review* 52 (2017): 19–42. https://doi.org/10.1016/j.cpr.2016.11.007.

ENDNOTES

GRATITUDE, BALANCE & ENERGY IN MOTION

1. Rebecca Alexander, Oriana R. Aragón, Jamila Bookwala, Nicolas Cherbuin, Justine M. Gatt, Ian J. Kahrilas, Niklas Kästner, et al., "The Neuroscience of Positive Emotions and Affect: Implications for Cultivating Happiness and Well-being," *Neuroscience and Biobehavioral Reviews* 121 (2021): 220–49. https://doi.org/10.1016/j.neubiorev.2020.12.002.

Lightning Source UK Ltd.
Milton Keynes UK
UKHW020336020922
408195UK00003B/315